THE DIRECT ANTERIOR APPROACH TO THE HIP

Michael Nogler, MD, MA, MSc

Department of Orthopaedic Surgery
Medical University
Innsbruck, Austria

HSC Press

ABOUT THE HOMER STRYKER CENTER

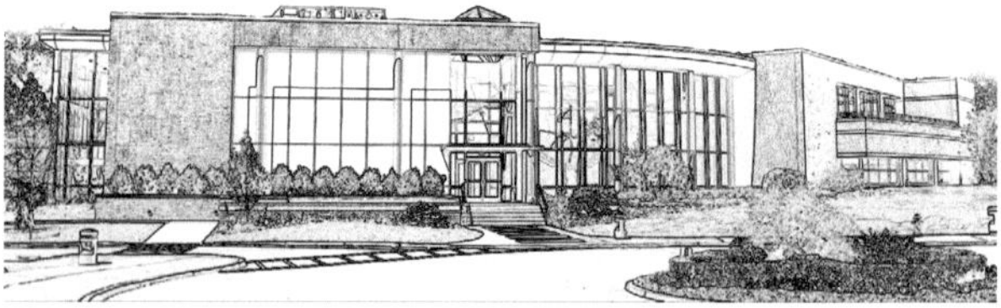

The Homer Stryker Center is dedicated to improving patient outcomes through education and research and works with an internationally recognized faculty to develop exceptional educational material using modern education technologies. The Center offers courses in orthopaedic bioskills and surgical simulation, as well as didactic education and discussion groups.

The HSC Press publishes course materials for the Homer Stryker Center.

HomerStrykerCenter®

HSC Press

Mahwah, New Jersey

ISBN 10: 0-9839-1514-8
ISBN 13: 978-0-9839151-4-0

ABOUT THE AUTHOR

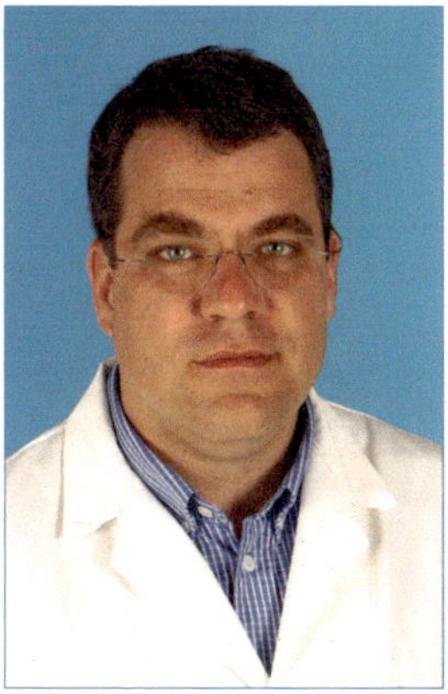

Michael Nogler, M.D., M.A., M.Sc.

Dr. Nogler is a graduate of the Medical University in Innsbruck, Austria and completed his post-graduate training at the University Hospital of Innsbruck, Department of Orthopaedics. He specializes in adult reconstruction with a focus on minimally invasive procedures and computer assistance.

In addition to being Vice Chairman of the Department of Orthopaedic Surgery at the Medical University of Innsbruck, Dr. Nogler is also Chairman of the Unit of Experimental Orthopaedics. He was appointed full professor of Experimental Orthopaedics in February, 2009.

Dr. Nogler created the Innsbruck Orthopaedic Training Centre, a leading educational facility in which more than 900 surgeons from 32 countries have been trained in the technique of the minimally invasive direct anterior approach to the hip.

CONTENTS

Introduction

The surgical approach for total hip arthroplasty via the interval between the tensor fasciae latae and the rectus femoris muscles has been in use for several decades.[1-3] Many authors have utilized variations of the direct anterior approach and have published their experience.[1, 2, 4, 5] Yet, this approach has not become a widely used standard approach to hip arthroplasty, like the posterior approach or variations of the lateral approach, largely due to lack of familiarity with the surgical technique.

With evolution of minimally invasive surgery, the direct anterior approach has garnered more attention. Human anatomy has provided us with two accessible intermuscular pathways to the hip joint, the interval between the tensor fasciae latae and gluteus medius muscles (Watson-Jones interval) and the interval between the tensor fascia latae and sartorius and rectus (direct anterior interval). Although both intervals are intermuscular, thedirect anterior interval has the advantage of also being truly internerval, as all the muscles located medially to that interval are supplied by the femoral nerve, and all the muscles located laterally are supplied by the superior gluteal nerve. This advantage makes the direct anterior interval the natural choice for a hip arthroplasty procedure that aims to spare the muscles and potentially reduce invasiveness overall.

Several techniques have been developed in recent years to utilize the direct anterior approach for muscle sparing total hip arthroplasty.[6-10] These techniques require a short skin incision and provide maximal protection to the structures underneath the skin. The technique that will be described in this book is one that was developed in Innsbruck, Austria and is now in use by many centers worldwide as increasing numbers of surgeons are choosing the direct anterior approach as their standard of care. This technique does require a set of specialized instruments but does not require a traction table, although one can be used if desired.[10-13]

As with all surgical procedures, it is natural for a surgeon who starts using a new surgical technique to develop variations of it over time in order to adapt the technique to his environment or specific needs. To simplify the teaching process, the technique has been standardized, and only a few possible variations are mentioned.

A Brief History of the Direct Anterior Approach

The direct anterior approach to hip replacement is not a new procedure. It is widely believed to be based on Hueter's anterior incision, which dates back to the 1880's.[14]

In 1917 Dr. Smith-Petersen first introduced his anterior technique for approaching the hip to address congenital hip reductions, with further writings published in 1931 and 1949.[3] He stressed correctly exposing the acetabulum[15] and devised his namesake approach during his internship in Massachusetts in 1916, at which time he suggested to a surgeon there had to be a better way to perform this procedure. The surgeon told him to find one, so he found a better way to improve the exposure of the head and neck of the femur; however, the acetabulum itself remained inaccessible. Smith-Petersen's approach was presented by Dr. Elliot G. Brackett at the American Orthopaedic Association meeting and was well received. In 1935, Dr. Smith-Petersen updated the approach to access the acetabulum, and for a number of years this newer approach was used commonly.[16] The anterior approach for total hip arthroplasty (THA) was first used by Dr. Robert Judet in 1947 as a modification of the Smith-Petersen approach for

THA.[17] Three years later, Drs. Judet and Judet introduced their version of the anterior approach to the hip in an article for the Journal of Bone and Joint Surgery (British) published in 1950.[18] In response to Whitman's technique, which was showing low patient success, the doctors Judet determined that the replacement of the femoral head would provide the patient with more stability.[17] The Judets preferred the anterior approach because when using this method, the hip joint presented closer to the skin than with other approaches. The Judets performed surgery on a table designed by Dr. Henri Judet. Judet used an orthopedic table with indirect traction applied to both feet, because traction applied to the lower limbs combined with traction and simultaneous external rotation and hyperextension in the hip joint of the treated limb facilitated hip joint dislocation.

In 1966, Dr. Heinz Wagner began clinical trials using the anterior approach for hip surface replacement surgery.[19] Dr. Wagner performed this procedure with the patient in the supine position. One of the most important features of Dr. Wagner's technique was that the bone stock remained protected, which allowed for a later procedure if necessary.

Drs. Terry Light and Kristaps Keggi introduced their version of the direct anterior technique at the American Academy of Orthopaedic Surgeons in 1979.[2] Since then, the anterior approach has been used by Keggi in over 7,000 patients.[20] In their 1980 article on the first 104 hips operated on with the direct anterior approach, Light and Keggi stated that the anterior approach includes an easy exposure to the hip joint and a low morbidity rate.[2] Additional reported benefits included shorter operating room time and less blood loss, which reduced the need for transfusions. It was noted also that patients were walking sooner, and no deaths were reported. Two of the patients suffered numbness in the lateral femoral cutaneous nerve due to the way the procedure was first performed. As a result, the authors decided to split the tensor fascia latae muscle, after which no post operative numbness was reported.[2]

In their 1993 article, Drs. Keggi, Huo and Zatorski reported on their first 1,000 total hip arthroplasties performed using the anterior method.[21] They made a curved incision and exposed the tensor fascia lata. The incision crossed an "internervous line". Medially retracted muscles were stimulated by the femoral nerve, and laterally retracted muscles were innervated by the superior gluteal nerve. Several different cup and stem designs were used during the ten-year period when the total hip arthroplasties were performed. Complication rates, including dislocation and infection, were reportedly low. The authors reported a 0.2% infection rate in their cases. Similar to the study reported on in 1980, the authors noted a low rate of thromboembolic disease in their patients following the anterior approach procedures.[20]

Dr. Joel Matta introduced his version of the direct anterior approach to the United States in 1996.[5, 22] Dr. Matta advocated performing the surgery on an orthopaedic (traction) table. Prior to 2002, Dr. Matta performed the anterior approach using the Smith-Petersen technique, but he currently uses a modification of the anterior approach as performed by Judet and Judet. Dr. Matta refers to the technique as Anterior Approach – Total Hip Arthroplasty (AA-THA) and has reported on close to 1,000 procedures using this method.[5]

At the University Hospital of Innsbruck, a direct anterior approach technique based on the concept of minimal muscle trauma was introduced by Dr. Rachbauer, Dr. Krismer, and Dr. Nogler.[23] In 2006, Dr. Michael Nogler introduced a specific instrument for use with a minimally invasive direct anterior approach (DAA).[13] The double offset broach handle (lateral and anterior offset) reduces the need for leverage of the proximal femur for preparation of the femoral canal. The Innsbruck technique is performed using a standard surgical table. In his 2008 article, Dr. Nogler reports on the effects of using navigation in cup positioning. In a cadaveric study, no navigation was used to ream the acetabulum and implant the cup in half of the specimens. The Stryker Hip Navigation system was used on the remaining group of specimens. It was determined that use of navigation can allow for placement of the cup during the anterior approach procedure.[8]

The Innsbruck technique is also used in the United States. In their 2008 article, Drs. Hozack and Klatt compare patients operated on using the DAA and the direct lateral approach. Although there were no significant differences in incision length, hospital stay, pain or blood loss, time to walking with a cane for DAA patients was reported at 2.4 weeks while direct lateral patients time to walking with a cane was reported at 3.7 weeks.[24] The authors also believe that the use of a second incision when performing the DAA is not necessary. In his 2008 paper, Dr. Tim Lovell advocates for performing the anterior approach on a standard operating table.[10] The author's list of benefits to using the anterior approach include not needing a member of the OR staff to move the leg during surgery and the ease of being able to check for stability, leg length and range of motion.

Why the Direct Anterior Approach?

The goal of the DAA is to be less invasive in THA and, as much as possible, to avoid muscle trauma. The anatomy of the hip joint provides only two portals that allow for direct access to the hip between the muscles and muscle groups. The first is the anterior portal between the sartorius and tensor (DAA). The second is the lateral portal between the tensor and the gluteus medius (Watson-Jones). Both portals can be and are used for total hip arthroplasty. The disadvantage of the latter is that, although it is intermuscular, it is not truly internerval.

The branches of the superior nerve cross the Watson-Jones portal a few centimeters proximally to the tip of the greater trochanter and are at risk of being damaged during surgery. Conversely, the direct anterior interval is intermuscular and truly internerval. All the medial muscles are supplied by the femoral nerve and the lateral muscle group is supplied by the superior gluteal nerve. No motor nerves are in the portal itself. Therefore, we choose to utilize the direct anterior intermuscular internerval portal for our minimally invasive technique.

When starting with something new it can be exciting to actually find out that this "new" thing is not really new. As we explained in our history section, the direct anterior approach is not only a well-established approach for accessing the hip joint and pelvis but is also well-established for use in total hip arthroplasty. Although we might have helped bring renewed popularity to this approach by focusing on its evident minimal invasiveness, it is and always has been a standard approach to THA.

Anatomic Considerations

The direct anterior approach utilizes the interval between tensor fasciae latae and sartorius as well as the rectus femoris **(Figure 1)**. It is, like the Watson-Jones interval (between tensor and gluteus medius), one of the two truly intermuscular intervals. But unlike the Watson-Jones interval, it is also truly internerval because all the muscles located medially to the interval are supplied by the femoral nerve, and all muscles located laterally are supplied by the superior gluteal nerve.

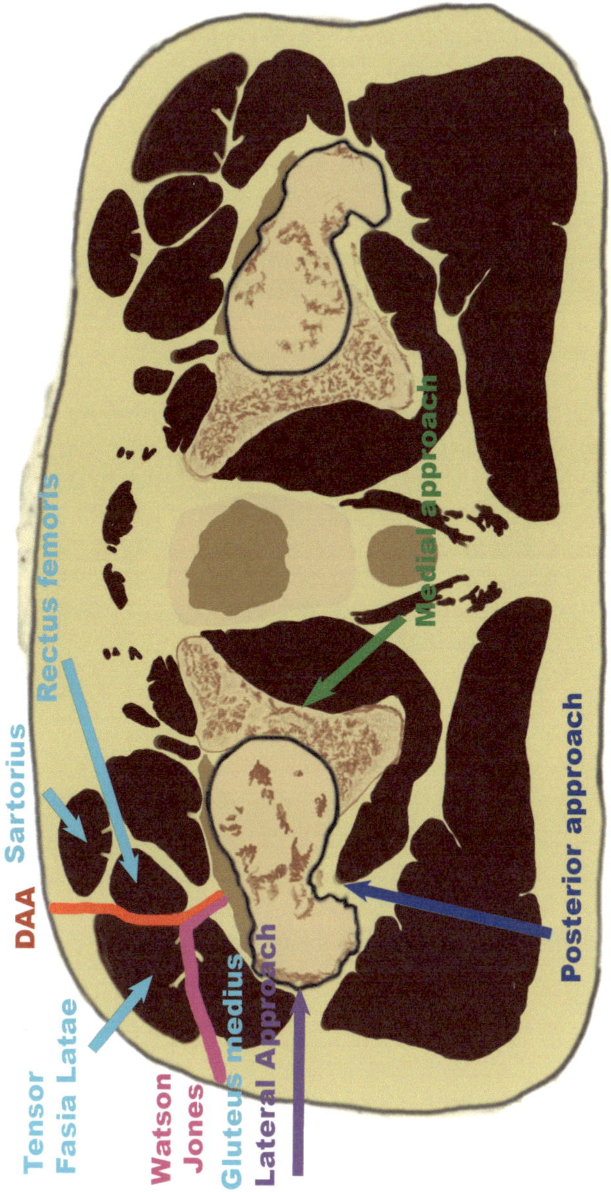
Tensor
Fasia Latae
DAA
Sartorius
Rectus femoris
Watson
Jones
Gluteus medius
Lateral Approach
Medial approach
Posterior approach

Figure 1

The superior gluteal nerve crosses the Watson-Jones interval about 4cm proximally to the tip of the greater trochanter. Damage of these branches could lead to degeneration of the tensor muscle **(Figure 2)**.

The anterior superior iliac spine is the center of a coordinate system for the orientation of the skin incision. It is extremely important that the anterior superior iliac spine (ASIS) always be accessible and palpable during the surgery. Note that the ASIS marks the most proximal point for a proximal extension of the incision without muscle detachment **(Figure 3)**.

In order to avoid any damage to the lateral femoral cutaneous nerve, the starting point of the skin incision is placed 1.5cm distally and 2 to 3cm laterally to the ASIS **(Figure 4)**. This situs preparation shows the superficial portion of the interval that is bordered by the sartorius and tensor. The rectus femoris is one layer deeper underneath the sartorius and forms the deep medial border of the interval.

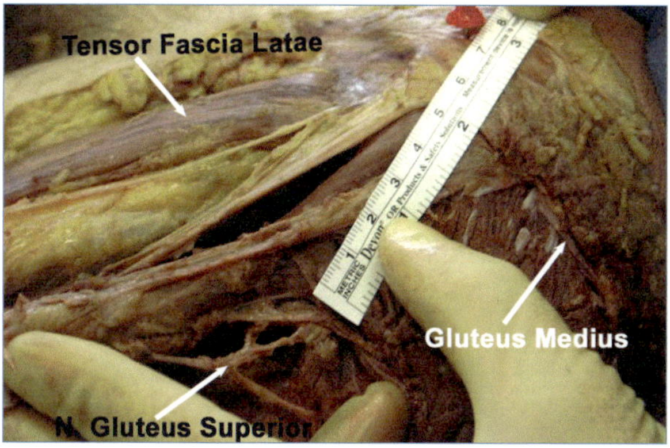

Figure 2

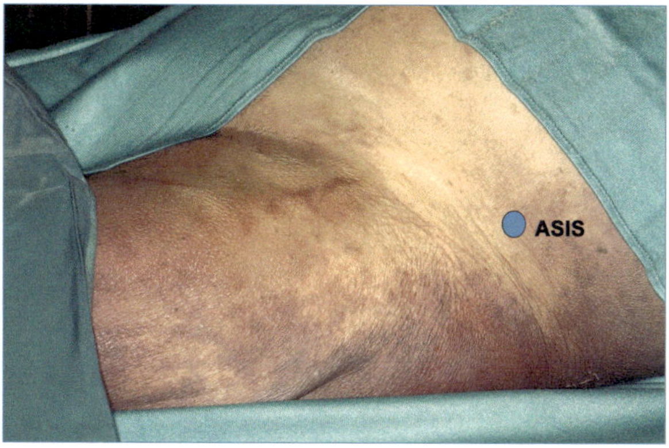

Figure 3

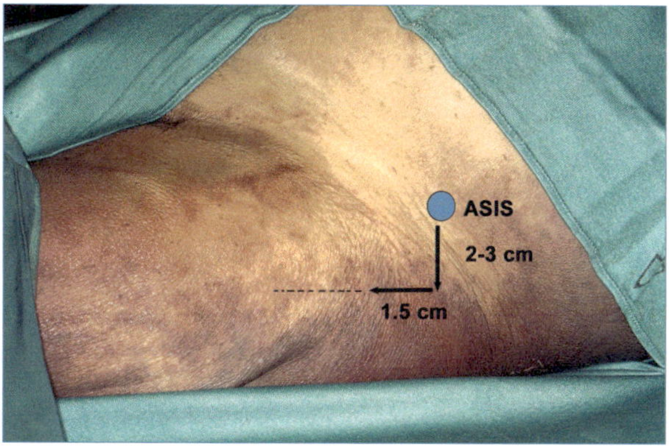

Figure 4

It is important to note the following:

- The sartorius and tensor originate from the ASIS area. A proximal extension of the approach beyond the ASIS requires detachment of the tensor from the ilium **(Figure 5)**.
- The tendinous portion of the origin of the tensor from the ilium and whether or not muscular detachment of the tensor is required and an incision in this area could be resutured successfully **(Figure 5)**.
- The lateral branch of the lateral femoral cutaneous nerve (LCFN) supplies an area of the skin located anterolaterally at the upper leg **(Figure 5)**.

Underneath the skin is a subcutaneous fat layer **(Figure 6)**.

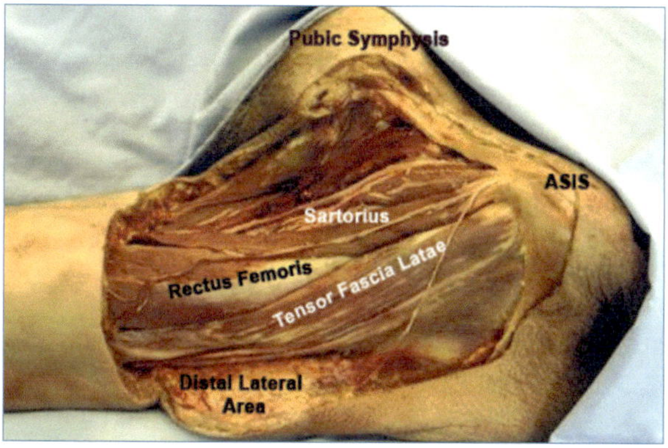

Figure 5

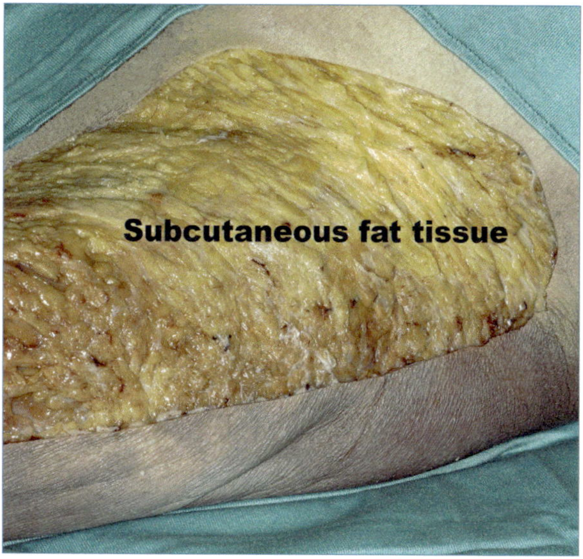

Figure 6

The main branches of the LCFN are medial to the ASIS. Note the perforating vessels at the dorsal border of the tensor and the white fascia that covers gluteus muscle dorsal to the tensor **(Figure 7)**.

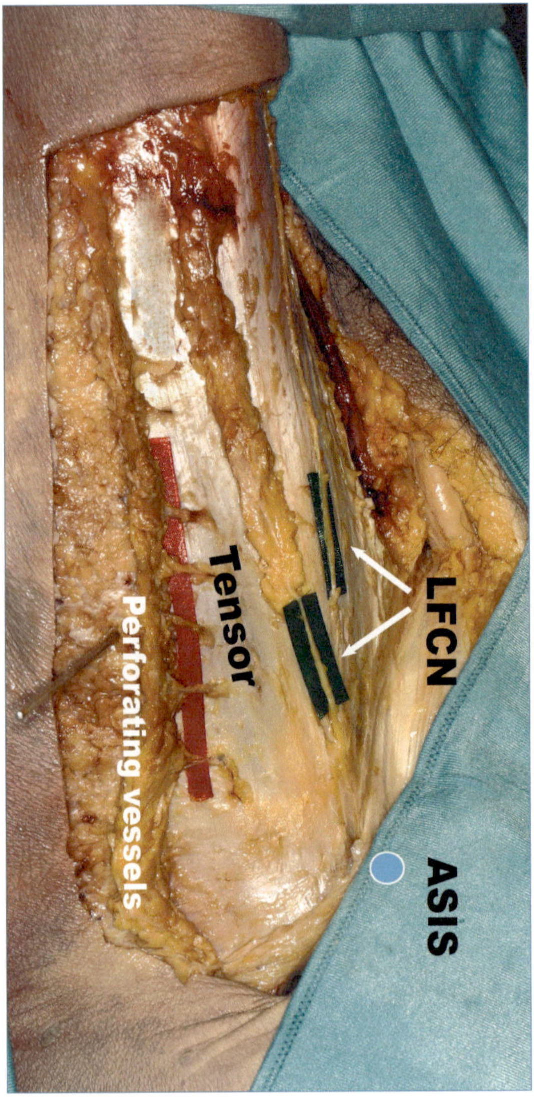

Figure 7

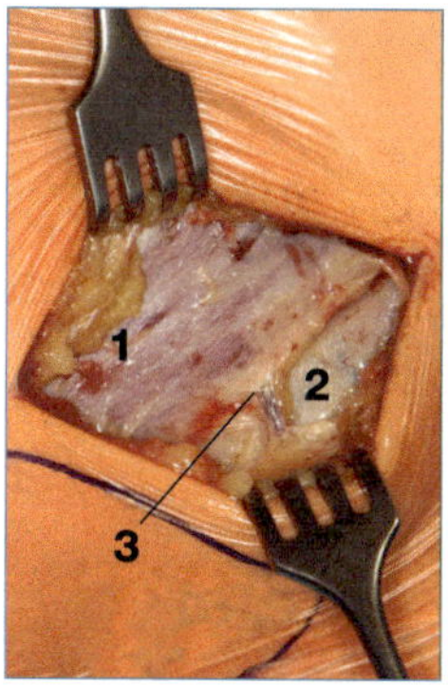

Figure 8

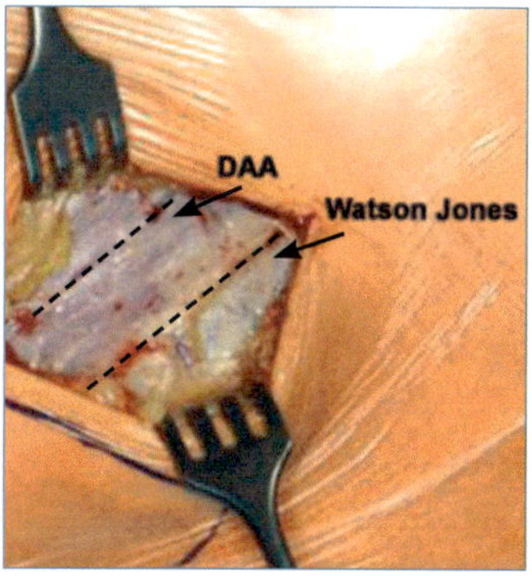

Figure 9

The anatomic dissection and the intra-operative view show the three anatomic landmarks that identify the tensor muscle **(Figure 8)**.

1. A red muscle covered by its fascia (TFL)
2. A white stronger fascia (iliotibial band) that covers the gluteus medius muscle
3. At least one perforating vessel at the dorsal border of the TFL

From this skin incision the Watson-Jones interval as well as the DAA interval can be reached **(Figure 9)**. The main branches of the LFCN are located medially to and at the level of the ASIS. In order to avoid any damage to them or their perineural tissue, the fascia of the tensor muscle is split at the lateral aspect and can be separated from the muscle fibers. The DAA interval can be reached underneath the fascia **(Figure 10a, 10b)**.

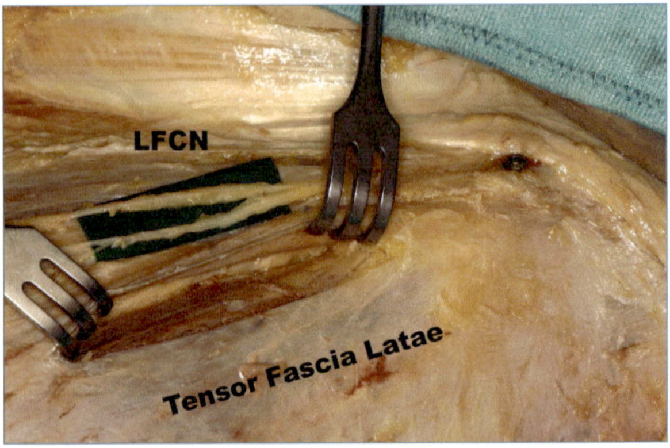

Figure 10a

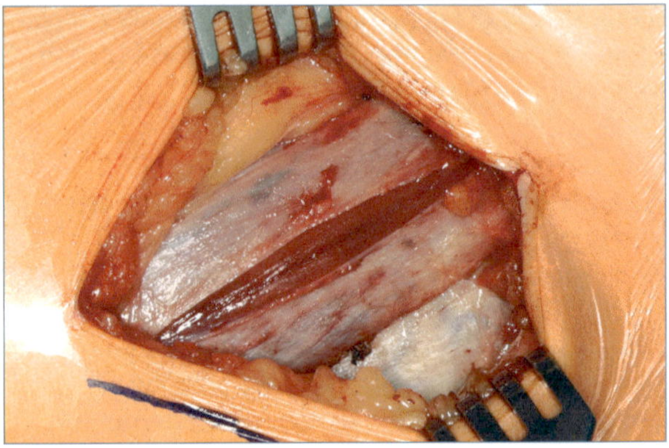

Figure 10b

In the exposed interval, a septum covers a vascular bundle. This septum has to be split in order to expose the vessels **(Figure 11)**.

The iliotibial band has a deep layer of fibers that originate from a point located distally and laterally and insert proximally and medially into the ventral hip joint capsule and the fascia of the sartorius, rectus, and vastus muscles **(Figure 12)**.

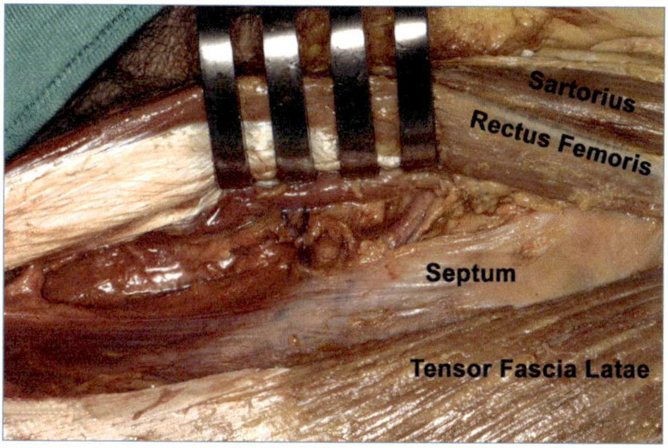

Figure 11

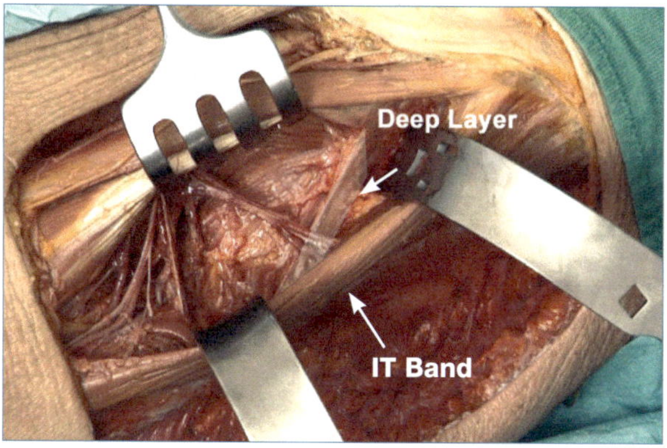

Figure 12

Note that the ascending branches are crossing the femoral neck proximal to the lateral vastus **(Figure 13)**. Branches of the femoral nerve, supplying the lateral vastus are crossing the femur distally to the lesser trochanter **(Figure 14)**.

The capsule has been removed and the reflected head of rectus is exposed. A major portion of the reflected head originates from the bony acetabular rim in normal hips and does not have to be incised for exposure. The portion of the reflected head which inserts into the hip capsule will be removed during the capsular resection. The head of the lateral vastus originates from the intertrochanteric line and forms a landmark for medial retractor placement and neck osteotomy **(Figure 15)**.

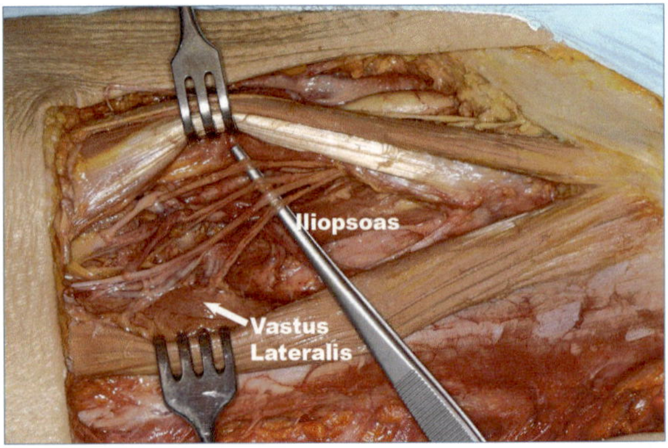

Figure 14

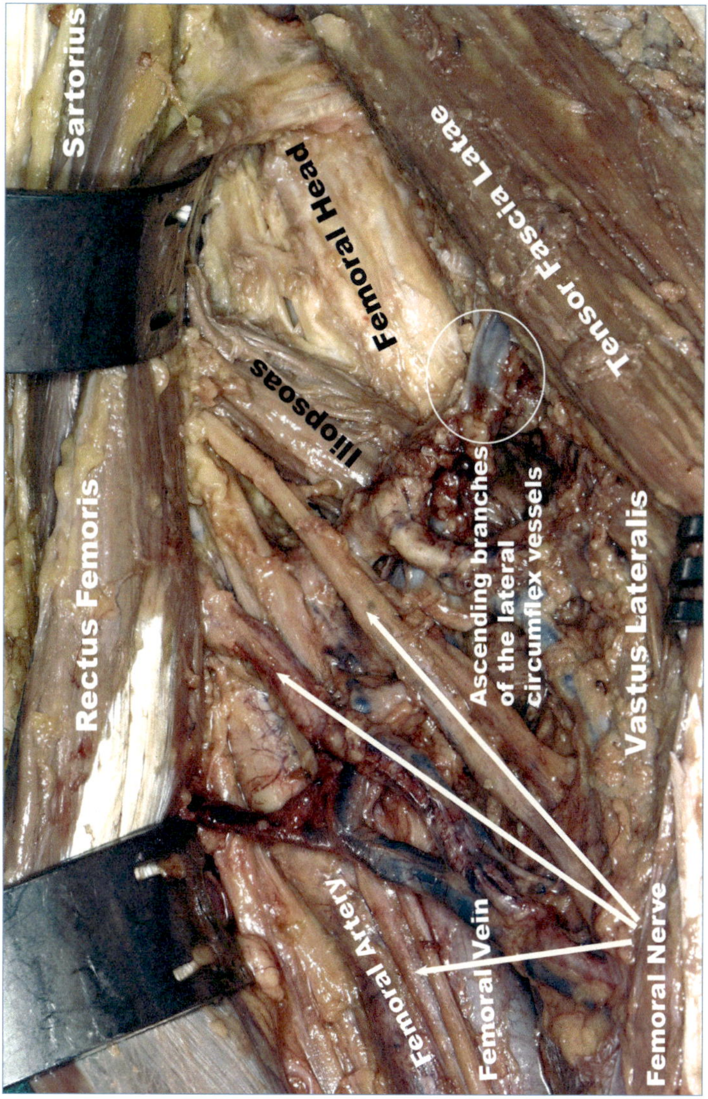
Sartorius
Femoral Head
Tensor Fascia Latae
Iliopsoas
Rectus Femoris
Ascending branches
of the lateral
circumflex vessels
Vastus Lateralis
Femoral Artery
Femoral Vein
Femoral Nerve

Figure 13

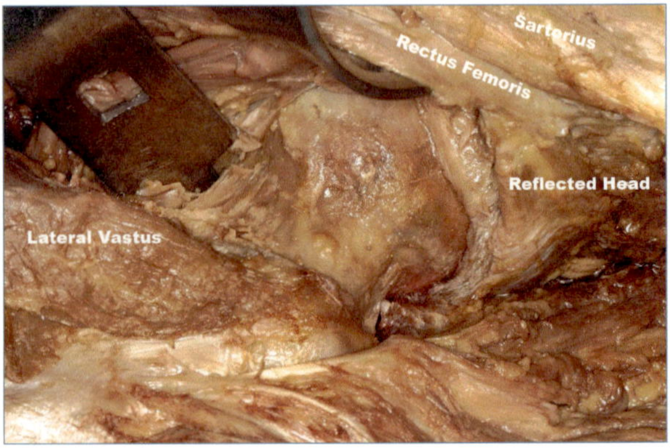

Figure 15

During the acteabular exposure it is helpful to place a ventral retractor underneath the sartorius, rectus, and iliopsoas. Orientation perpendicular to the ilioinguinal band avoids damage to the femoral neurovascular bundle **(Figure 16)**.

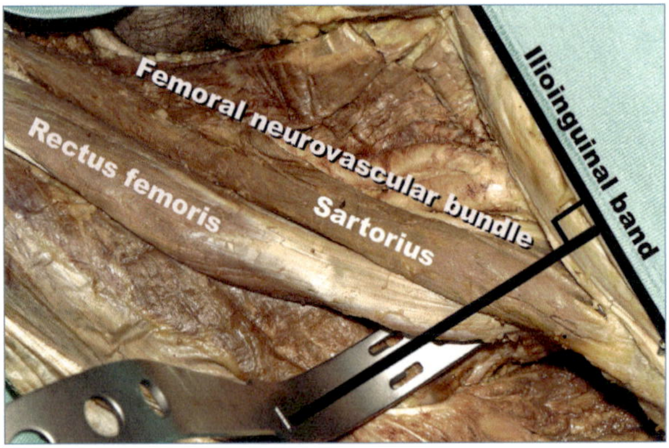

Figure 16

Remove the anterior capsule. Carefully detatch the capsule as distally as possible in order to expose the piriformis fossa and avoid the medius tendon and piriformis muscle. This cadaver exposure shows the attachment of the gluteus medius and the piriformis muscle **(Figure 17)**.

To describe relative orientation of the femoral cut surface and the acetabular rim, a coordinate system has been introduced, named, and numbered in clockwise direction. This coordinate system is also used to identify all portions of the capsule that are resected during the procedure **(Figure 18)**.

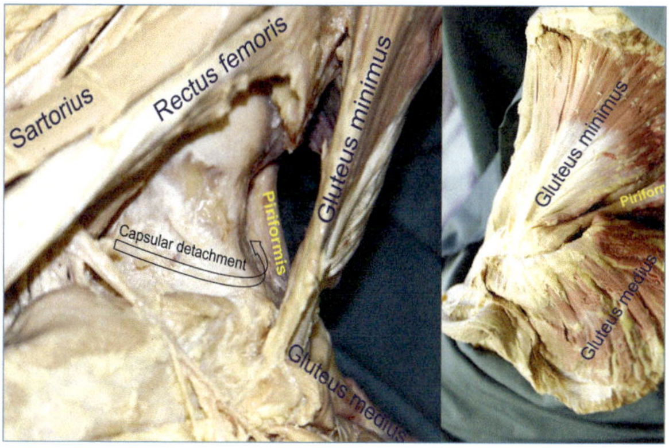

Figure 17

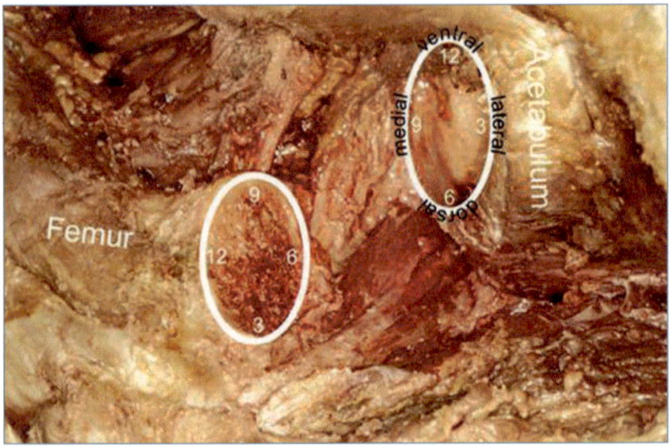

Figure 18

Located ventrally to the piriformis fossa is an anatomically nondescript area that we call "the saddle". It is the starting point for the osteotomy and needs to be carefully exposed and cleared of capsular tissue **(Figure 19)**.

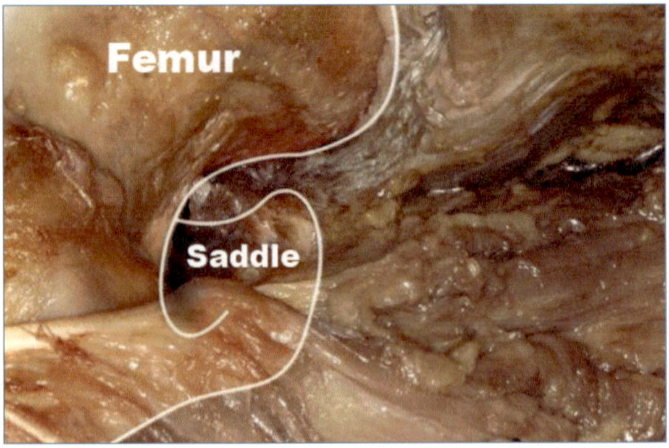

Figure 19

The small external rotators have been exposed from an anterior direction. The dorsal capsule and the dorsocapsular fat pad have been removed. Note the piriformis, the gemelli muscles, and the external obturator combine to form a joint tendon and usually cannot be distinguished individually at their later exposure during surgery **(Figure 20)**.

A posterior exposure shows the external rotators as well as the gluetal muscles.

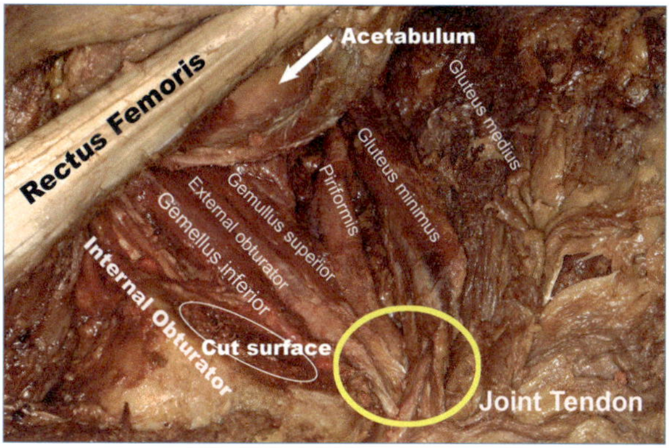

Figure 20

Note the distance of the sciatic nerve from the area of possible releases of the external rotators (yellow line) **(Figure 21)**.

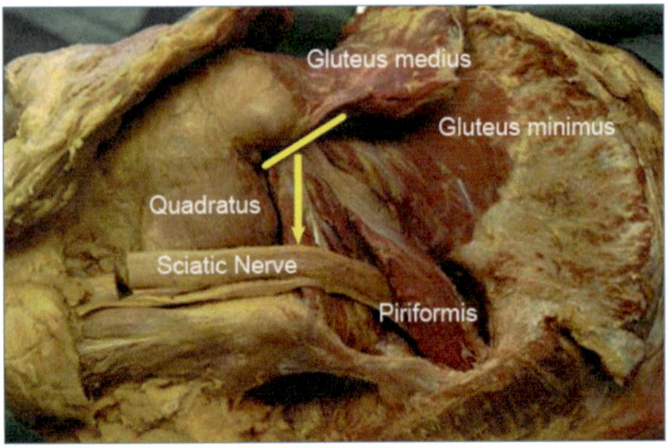

Figure 21

The "figure four" position of the operated leg gives an indication of the version of the stem. When the lower leg is brought into a horizontal plane, a perpendicular axis to that plane gives an estimation of the orientation of the retrocondylar line and thus indicates zero degrees of version. Anteversion of the stem can be achieved by rotating the implant against this axis **(Figure 22)**.

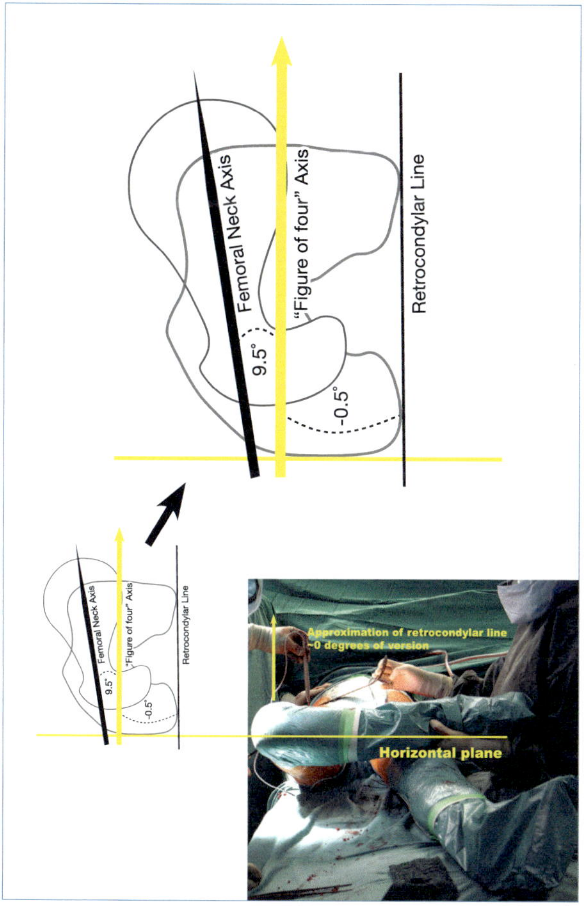

Figure 22. The figure four axis. (For more details, refer to Mayr E, et al. Acta Orthop. 2007;78:458-462.[25])

Patient Selection

The DAA is a standard approach to THA. Similar to other approaches, there will be easy cases, difficult ones, and many in between. When one first begins using the DAA, it is helpful to be able to identify the easier patients. Although there is no real algorithm to classify patients with regard to how easy or difficult their DAA THA will be, there are a few tips we can offer.

Muscles

A muscle sparing approach that exploits an intermuscular interval to replace hip joints is, by definition, dependent on muscle size and tone. In general, patients with strong, toned muscle are more difficult to operate on than those with flaccid muscle.

Relaxation

Muscle tension is also important. One's first few DAA cases preferably should be performed on fully relaxed muscles because that allows for better exposure of the femur.

BMI

The hip anterior portal is an area with a relatively small fat layer compared to lateral or posterior approaches. Hence, for many surgeons, the DAA is the approach of choice for a patient with a high BMI. Nevertheless, obese patients are more difficult to operate on no matter what approach is used and the size of the instruments, especially those with an offset, must be considered.

Femur Configurations

In general, varus hips are more difficult to operate on. This is true also for the DAA. Usually, a high collodiaphyseal (CCD) angle makes the surgery easier. Even more important is the absolute dimension of the neck. A long neck simply creates a larger distance between the cut surface of the femur and the acetabulum. In such patients, the tools can be introduced more easily.

Pelvis Configuration

The lateral distance of the anterior superior iliac spine (ASIS) from the center of rotation of the hip joint will give some estimation of the level of difficulty of the femoral exposure. Wide overhanging pelvises that reach far out laterally from the center of the hip are more difficult to operate on because the broach handle will be closer to the ASIS.

Contraindications

The DAA is a standard approach to the hip and is not limited to a certain type of case. Care should be taken in obese patients with moist areas and potential infections in the groin. Such areas must be avoided, and the skin incision should be placed more laterally. If this is not possible, a different approach should be considered.

Instrumentation

The DAA approach requires some specialized instrumentation. It is important to become familiar with the tools you will need to perform this surgical approach.

Retractors

Special retractors were designed with dual curves. The goal of this design is:

1. To reduce compression forces on soft tissue.
2. To lead the instrument out of the wound and maximize the wound opening.
3. To create an approximately 1 meter diameter workspace for the hands of the surgeon **(Figure 23)**.

Femoral Elevator

The femoral elevator, a posterior femoral retractor, was developed to improve the exposure of the proximal femur. The instrument is placed behind the greater trochanter at a 45° angle. The long teeth allow full support of the trochanteric bone and minimize the risk of trochanter fractures **(Figure 24)**. **Note:** Do not use this instrument as double prong retractor for acetabular exposure.

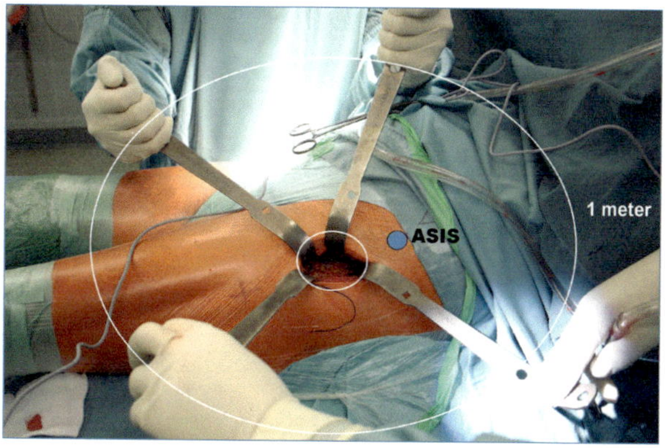

Figure 23

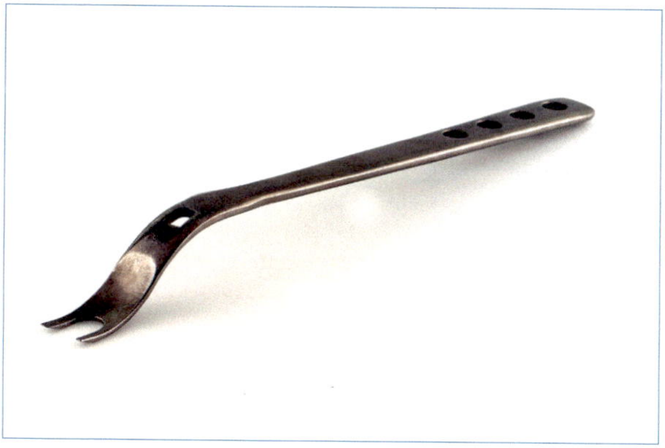

Figure 24

Standard Mueller Retractor

For acetabular exposure a standard Mueller retractor **(Figure 25a)**, or a curved acetabular retractor that also has two teeth, is especially helpful in facilitating acetabular exposure by pushing down the posterior and the proximal femur using a weight. Alternatively, a left or right curved acetabular retractor can be used **(Figure 25b)**. One of the two assistants can be replaced by a self retaining holding device that allows full retraction of soft tissue while holding the DAA retractors **(Figure 26a, 26b)**.

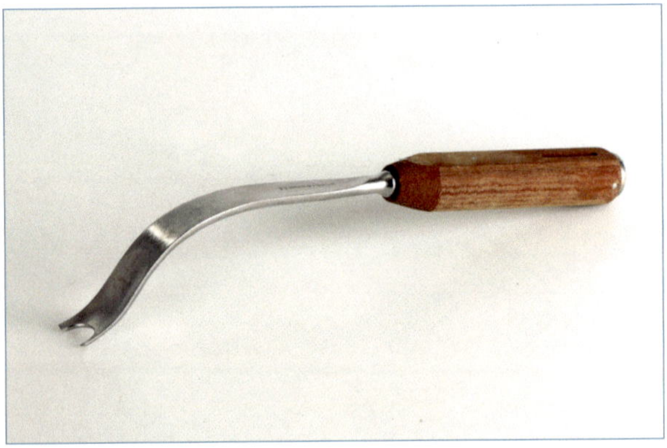

Figure 25a

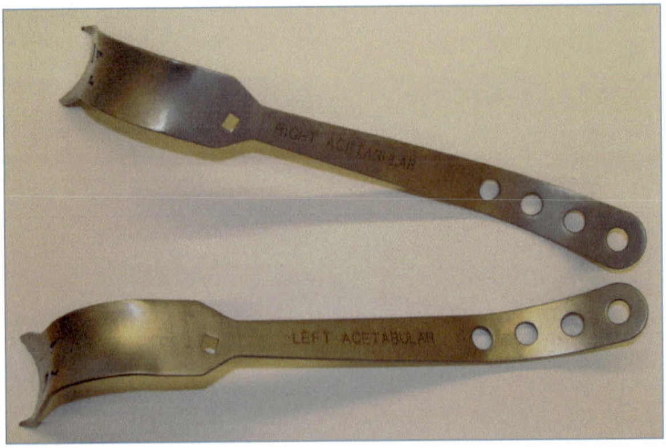

Figure 25b

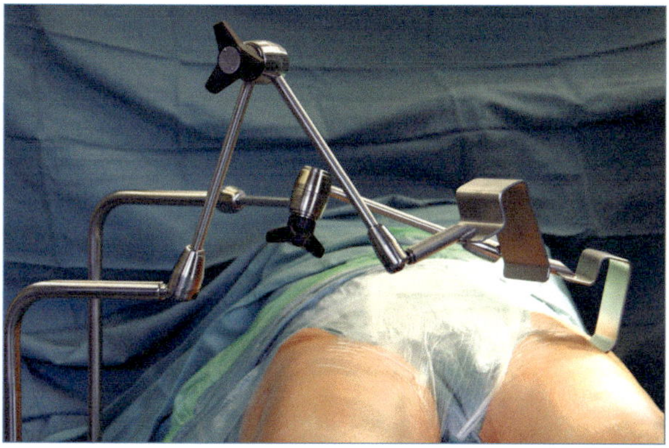

Figure 26a

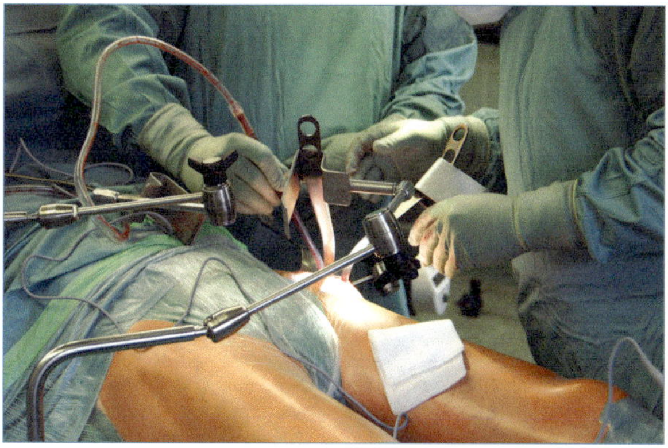

Figure 26b

Colorado Needle (Optional Device)

For cutting in a small wound, a device is suggested that does not require much force yet allows for precise soft tissue dissection. An electrocautery device, such as the Colorado Needle, is well insulated and is available with a 45° angulated tip **(Figure 27a, 27b)**.

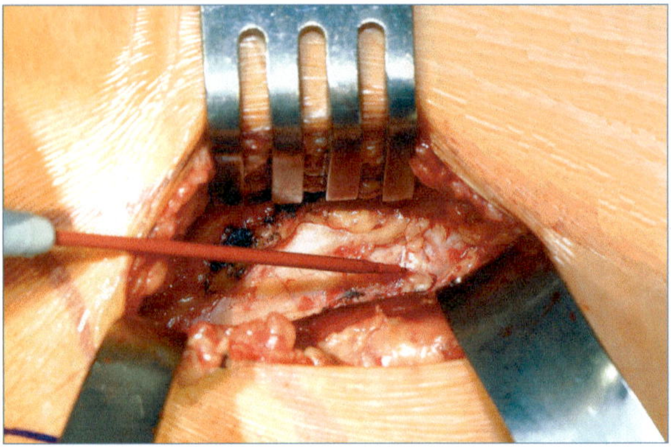

Figure 27a

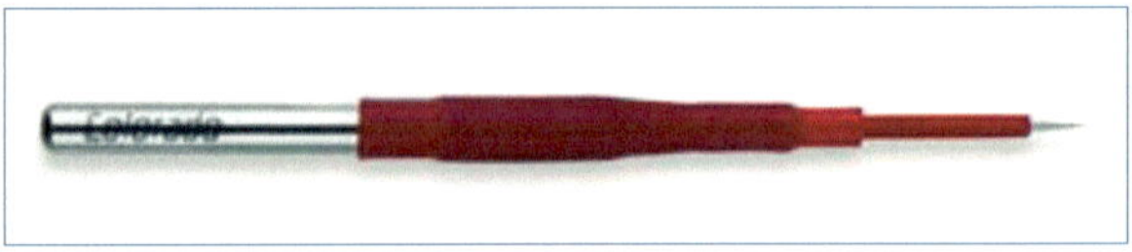

Figure 27b

Micro Saw

A small saw like the CORE micro saw (a), or a precision saw with an oscillating tip (b), is excellent for the osteotomy. These types of precision saws allow full visualization of the cutting process and help prevent soft tissue damage **(Figure 28a, 28b)**.

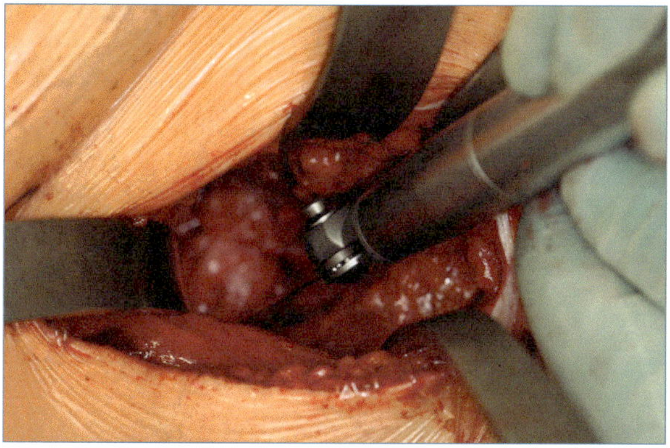

Figure 28a

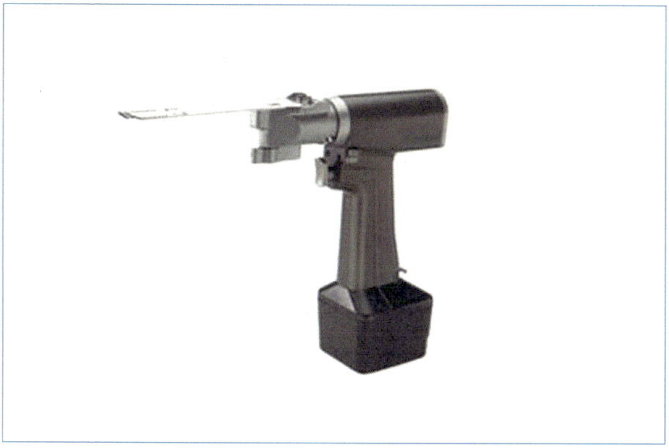

Figure 28b

Corkscrew

A standard corkscrew can be used to remove the femoral head **(Figure 29)**.

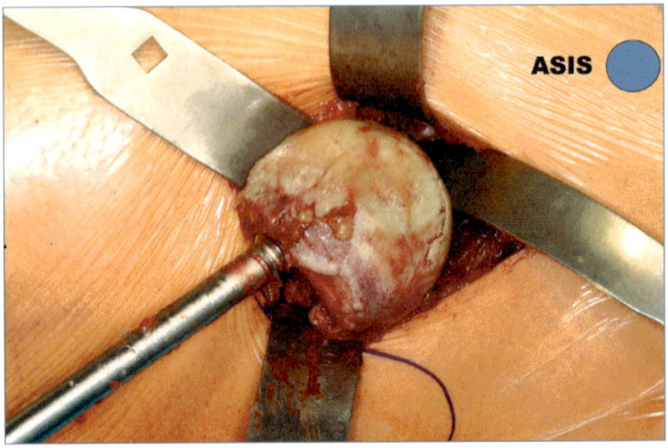

Figure 29

Double Offset Reamer

A double offset reamer handle allows for control of inclination and anteversion during reaming. The handle can be adjusted to accommodate left or right use **(Figure 30)**.

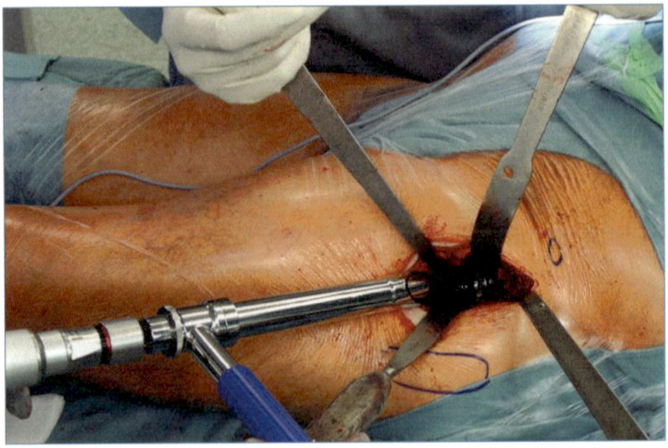

Figure 30

Curved Cup Impactor

For cup impaction a curved cup impactor is essential (a). The curved cup impactor also allows for introduction of either a ceramic or polyethylene liner into a seated cup (b). If a cup with screw holes is used, place the cluster of holes at the correct position on the curved cup impactor, because the handle cannot be rotated very much once inside the acetabulum **(Figure 31a, 31b)**.

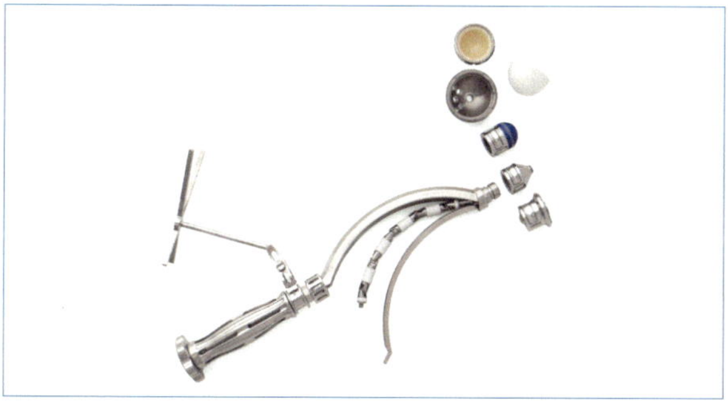

Figure 31a

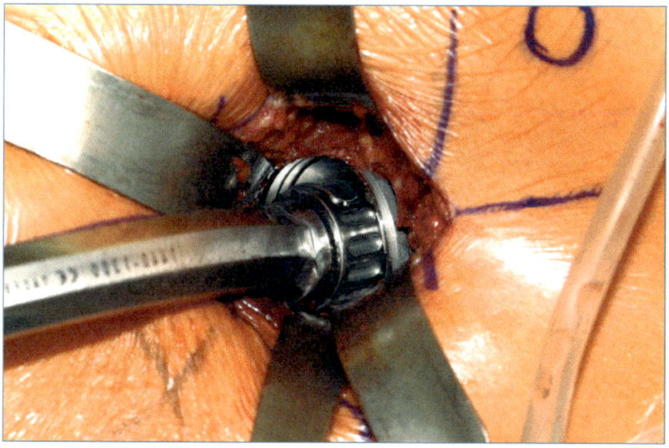

Figure 31b

Drill

A 90° drill allows for easy placement of the screws through the screw holes. Use either a screwdriver with a universal joint or a flexible screwdriver to place the screws **(Figure 32a, 32b, 32c)**.

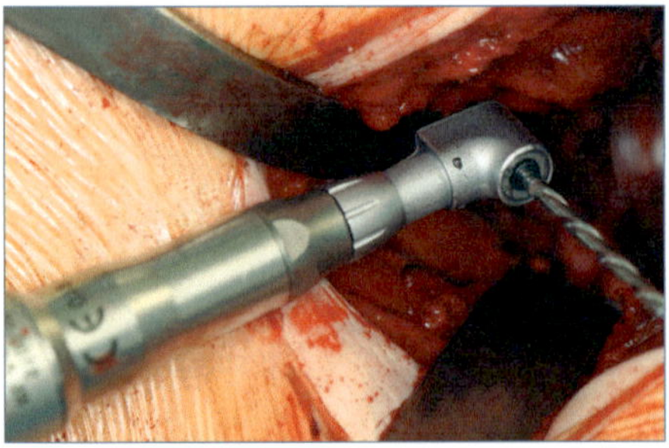

Figure 32a

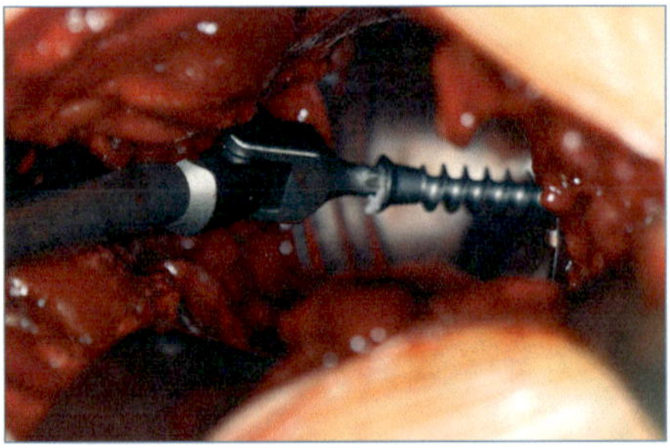

Figure 32b

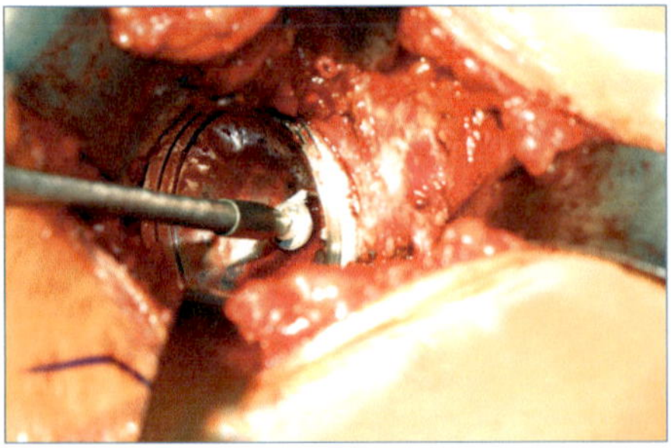

Figure 32c

Starter Broach

A proximal starter broach is used **(Figure 33)**.

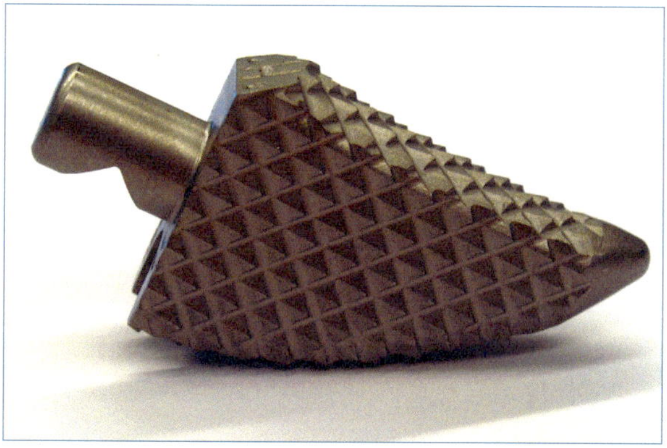

Figure 33

Broach Handle

The starter broach is mounted to the double offset broach handle and is used to shape the proximal femoral canal **(Figure 34)**.

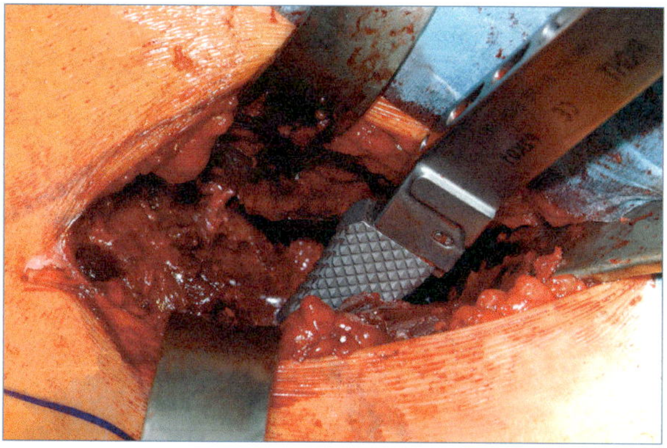

Figure 34

Double Offset Broach Handle

The double offset broach handle is the most important instrument for femoral preparation. It has both anterior and lateral offsets and comes in left and right versions **(Figure 35a, 35b)**.

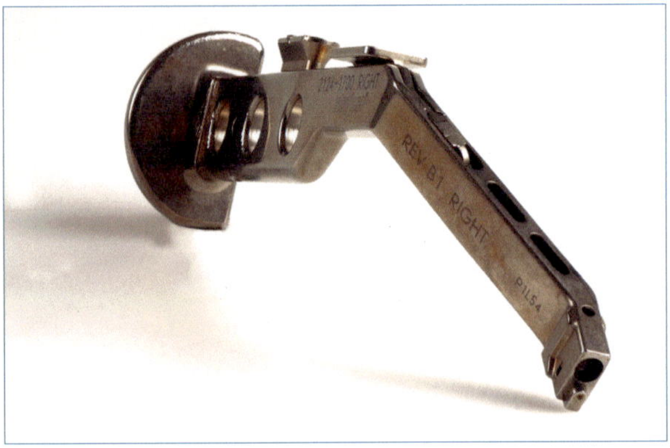

Figure 35a

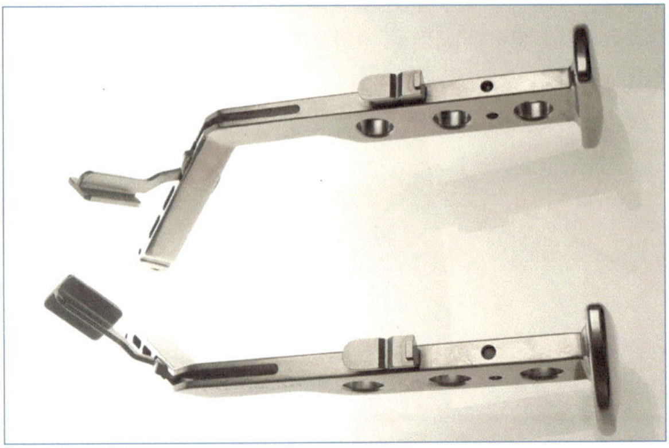

Figure 35b

Lighting

Visibility in a small wound is often reduced by insufficient lighting. Additional illumination can be facilitated by the use of head mounted lights as well as a light pipe system connected to a retractor **(Figure 36a, 36b, 36c)**.

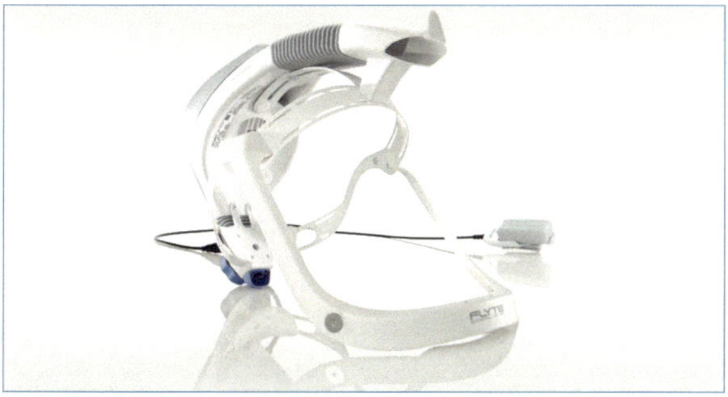

Figure 36a

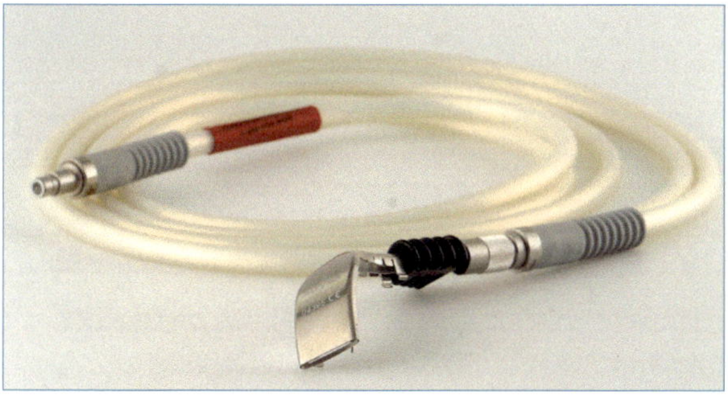

Figure 36b

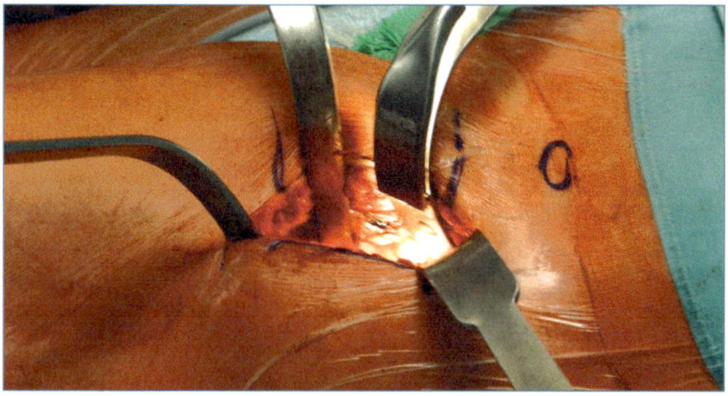

Figure 36c

Standard Angulated Curette

A major objective of this technique is to open up the femoral canal before broaching. A standard curved curette is used to perform the initial opening, to carve out the proximal cavity, and to remove debris during broaching **(Figure 37)**.

Note: Avoid using a straight instrument as this increases the risk of lateral perforation.

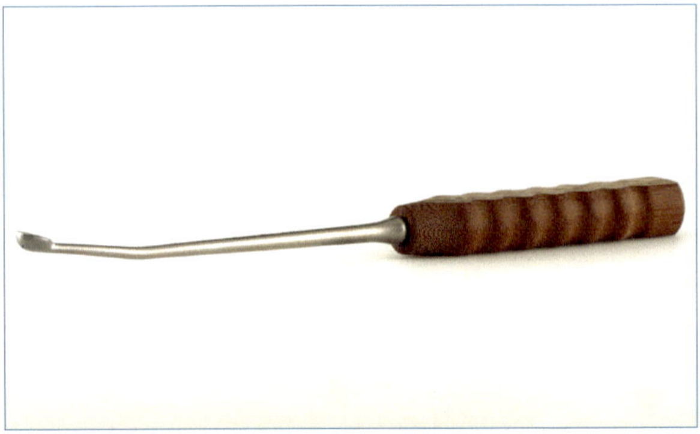

Figure 37

Direct Anterior Approach MIS Technique

The direct anterior approach (DAA) can be used to implant a standard total hip prosthesis using instruments designed specifically for minimally invasive surgery (MIS).

This technique allows direct, unimpeded access to the hip capsule through a single incision. The approach is made through an intermuscular and intervenous plane that spares tissue and leaves the gluteal muscles attached to the ilium.

Patient Preparation and Joint Exposure

Pre-operative Planning

Pre-operative planning aids in the selection of the appropriate implant style and size for the patient's hip pathology. Pre-operative X-ray analysis can be used to evaluate:

- Optimal femoral stem fit
- Prosthetic neck length
- Neck offset
- Acetabular component sizing
- Correct location of the osteotomy

Determination of probable implant style and size can facilitate operating room preparation by ensuring that the appropriate size selection is available. Anatomic anomalies that could prevent the intra-operative achievement of the established pre-operative goals may also be detected through such planning.

Patient Positioning

Place the patient in the supine position at the operating table. An optional table attachment opposite to the operated side (such as an arm board) allows for easier hyper abduction of the opposite leg during femoral exposure. Both legs are draped flexibly. Although only the operative leg needs to be sterilely draped, sterile draping of both legs may be helpful for the surgical exposure **(Figure 38)**.

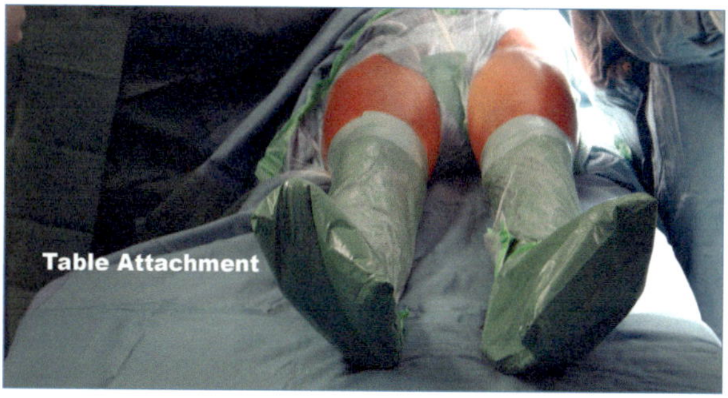

Figure 38

The Portal

Palpate the anterior superior iliac spine and the greater trochanter. The proximal starting point is found two finger breadths laterally and two finger breadths distally to the ASIS. The initial incision usually has a length of 6cm to 9cm. Observe that the location of the incision is located significantly more lateral than the original Smith-Petersen interval **(Figure 39)**.

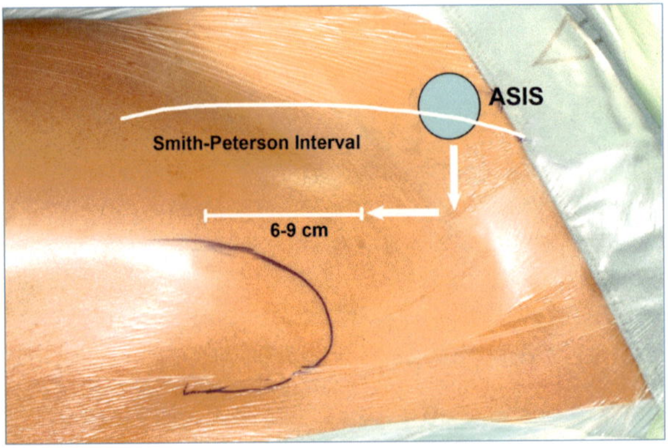

Figure 39

The LFCN is in the area of this approach. Placing the incision as described previously protects the nerve **(Figure 40)**.

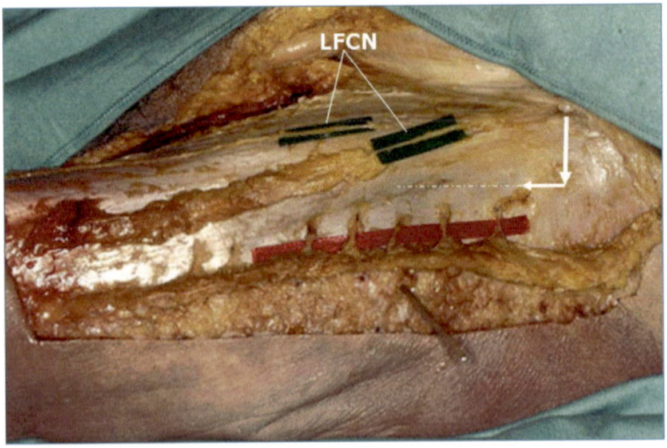

Figure 40

The anatomic dissection and the intra-operative view show the three anatomic landmarks that identify the tensor muscle **(Figure 41)**.

1. A red muscle covered by its fascia
2. A white stronger fascia (iliotibial band) that covers the gluteus medius muscle
3. At least one perforating vessel at the dorsal border of the muscle (needs to be cauterized)

Avoid cutting into the tensor fasciae latae (TFL) before precisely locating the correct portal. Use your index finger in proximal distal movements to palpate the interval between the TFL and sartorius. Note that the distance between the DAA interval and the interval medial to the sartorius is minimal **(Figure 42)**.

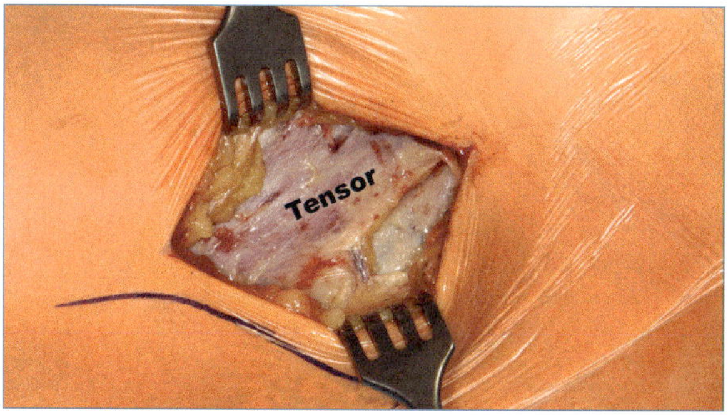

Figure 41

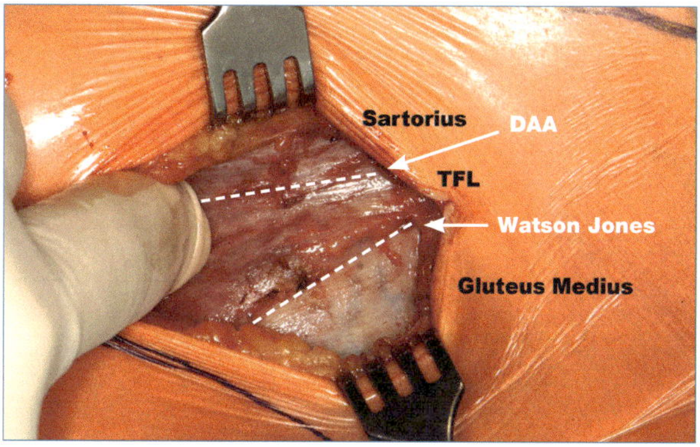

Figure 42

Exposure of the Joint

Use of Lateral Retractors

Sharply incise the fascia of the tensor at its mid-point in a medial to lateral direction. Dissect the fascia from the muscular fibers and perform the next steps strictly under the fascia. Gently pulling the TFL muscle fibers laterally beneath the TFL fascia easily reveals the Smith Petersen interval; this is identified as a fatty layer **(Figure 43a, 43b)**. Using your index finger, you can carefully explore the intermuscular interval and palpate the hip joint capsule **(Figure 44)**.

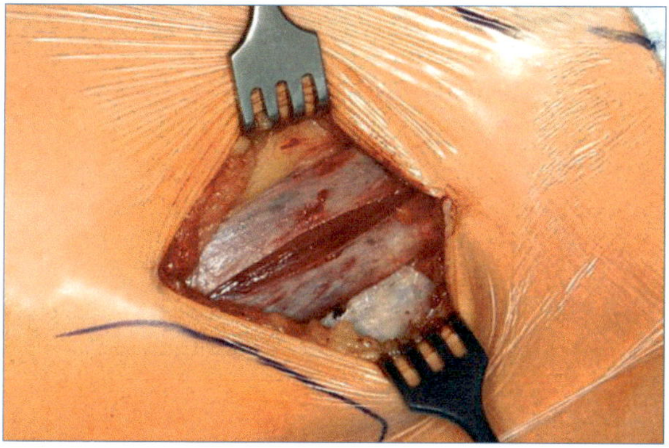

Figure 43a

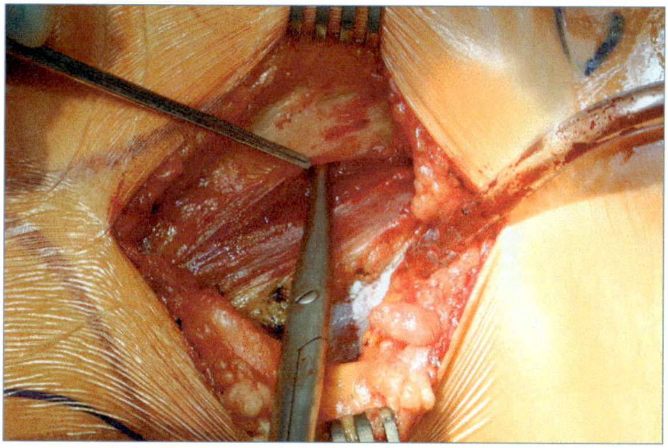

Figure 43b

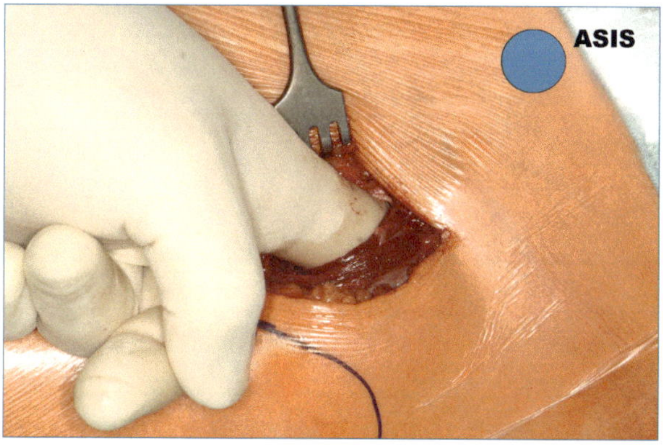

Figure 44

Place the first sharp or blunt (per surgeon preference) retractor (1) around the lateral or superior neck. Gentle pushing with your finger in this area prior to placing the retractor can identify the proper retractor location. Place the second sharp retractor (2) in the area of the greater trochanter. A rake or Hibbs retractor holds back the medial soft tissue **(Figure 45a, 45b, 45c)**. The ascending branches of the lateral circumflex vessels need to be identified and cauterized or ligated. These branches are variable in number **(Figure 46a, 46b)**.

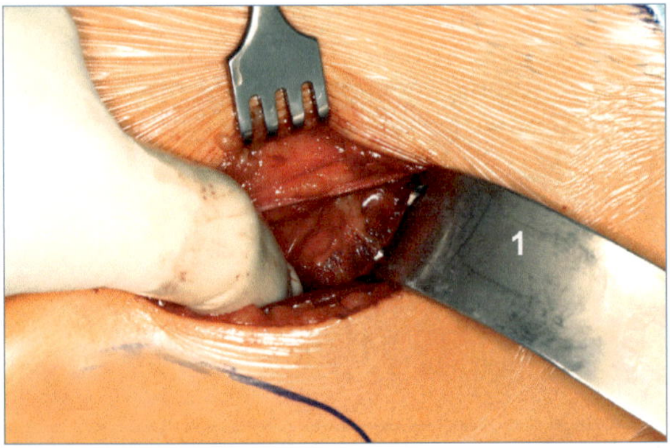

Figure 45a

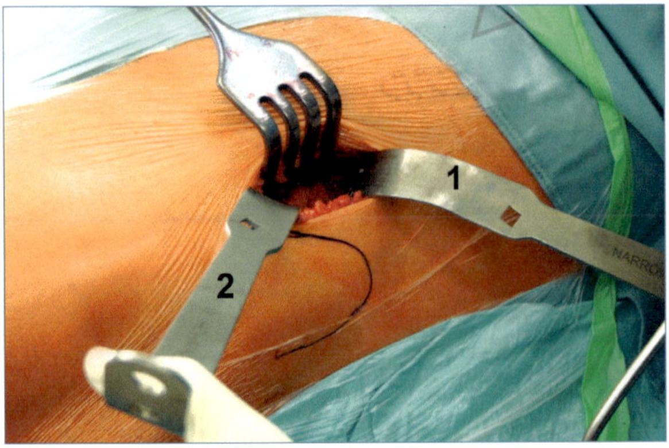

Figure 45b

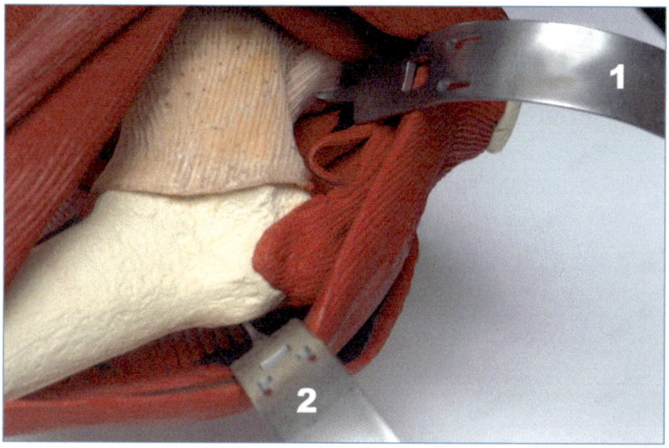

Figure 45c

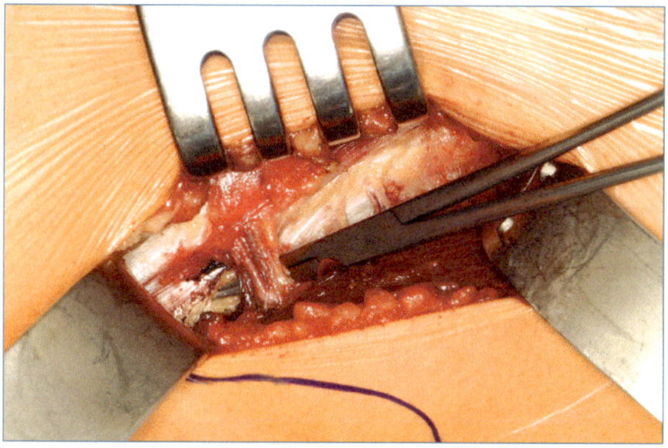

Figure 46a

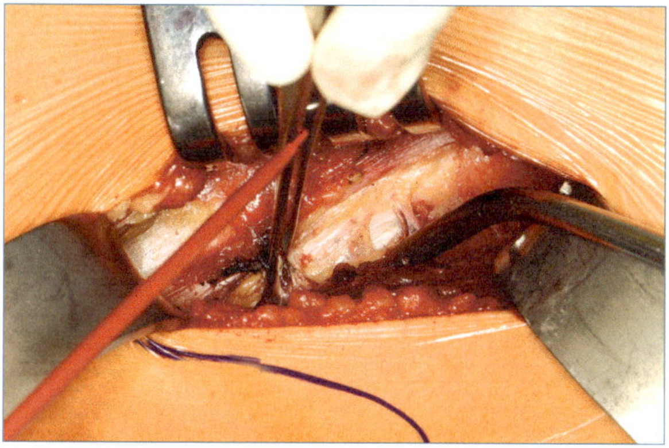

Figure 46b

Use of Medial Retractors

Once cauterized, the surgeon can incise a fascial layer between the rectus and the TFL. This layer is primarily formed by the deep layer of the ilioinguinal band. The fascial layer is cut with a Colorado Needle or bovie until the precapsular fat pad is visible. **(Figure 47a, 47b)**.

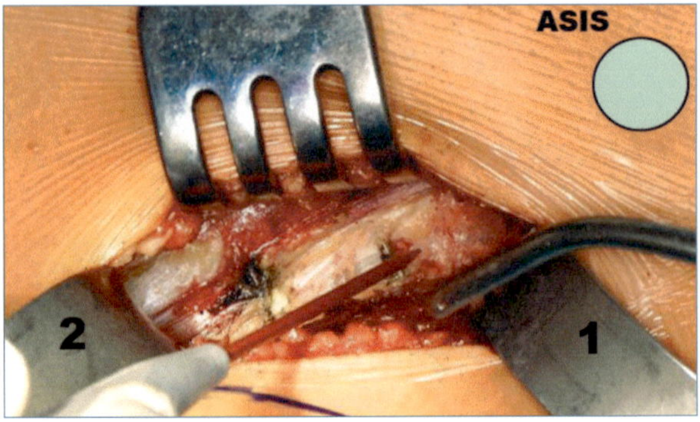

Figure 47a

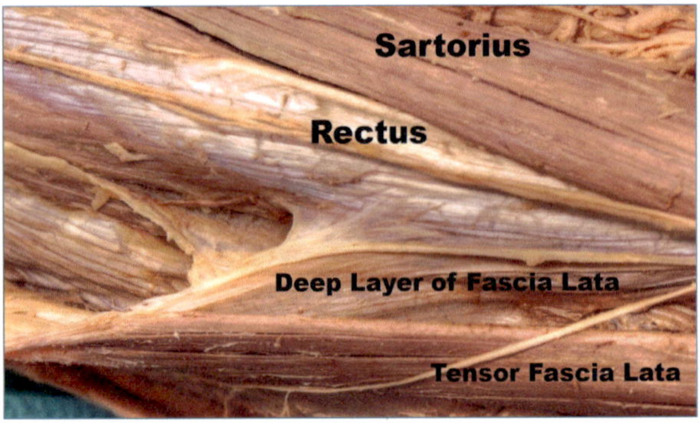

Figure 47b

The hip is flexed during this step. A "soft spot" which offers very little resistance can be palpated just proximally to the lateral vastus muscle. Blunt dissection with a finger or cobb can identify the proper location for the retractor. Stay in the precapsular fat pad. Cutting in to the fascia reveals the origin of the vastus lateralis and the precapsular fat pad. **(Figure 48a, 48b, 48c)**.

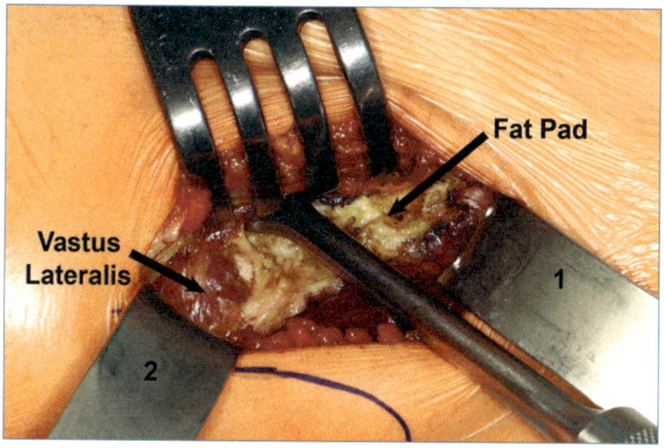

Figure 48a

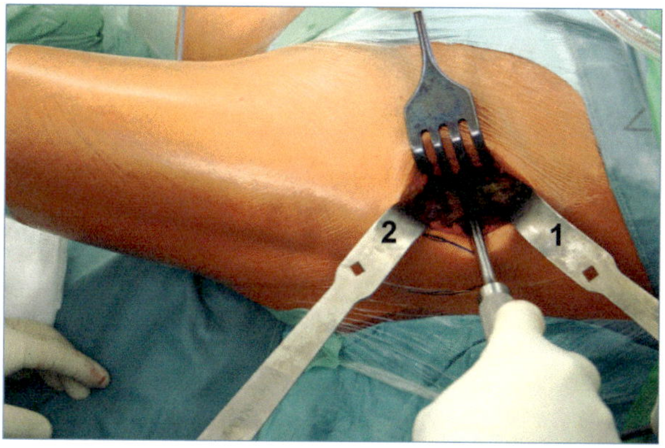

Figure 48b

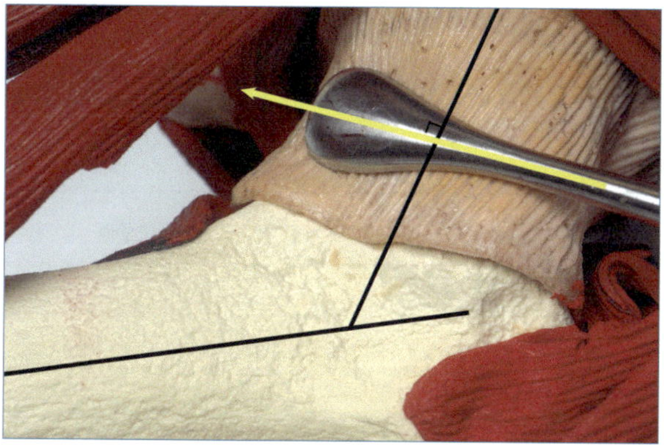

Figure 48c

Place another retractor (3) medially to the neck, thus retracting the rectus and sartorius. This can be either a sharp or blunt retractor **(Figure 49a, 49b)**.

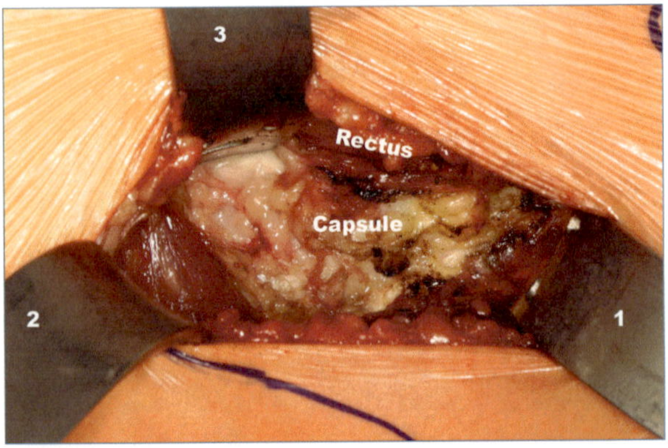

Figure 49a

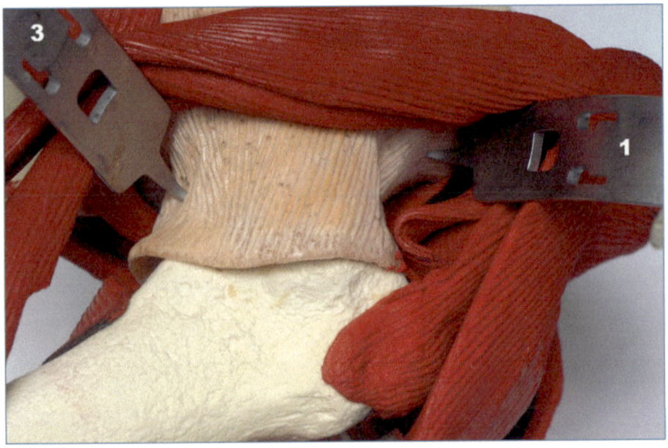

Figure 49b

The distal lateral retractor (2) can be removed for this step. After releasing the strong fascia under the rectus, the Cobb is used to prepare the space around the ventral rim of the acetabulum. The hip is flexed during this step **(Figure 50a, 50b, 50c)**.

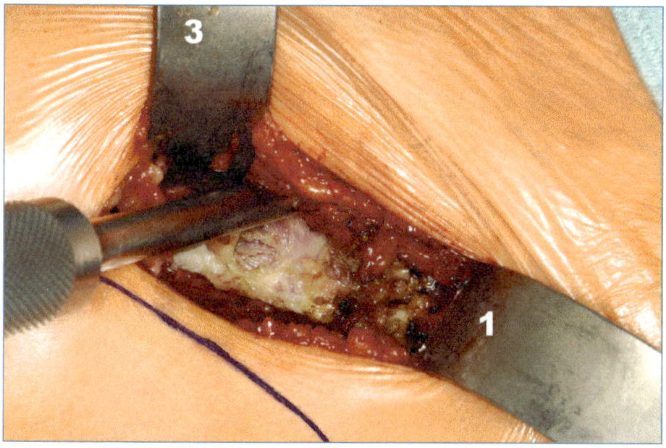

Figure 50a

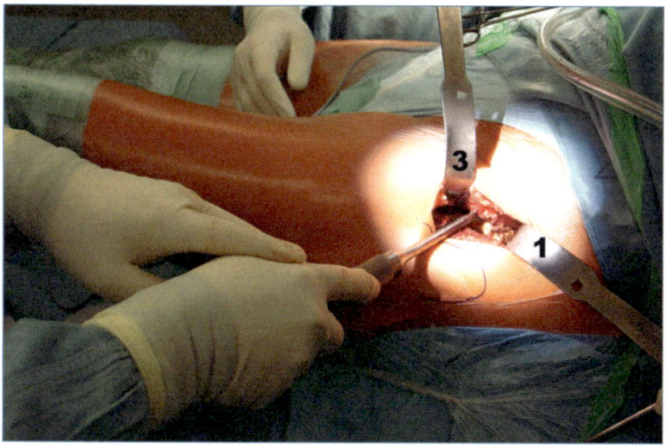

Figure 50b

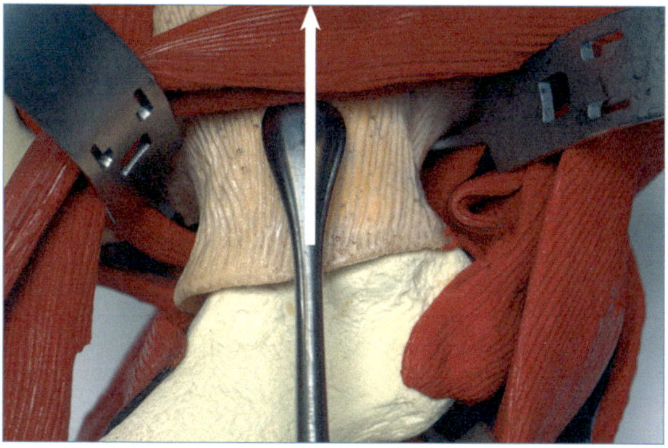

Figure 50c

A fourth sharp retractor (4) is placed around the ventral rim. A light attachment to this retractor can dramatically enhance visualization of the acetabulum. If necessary a further release of the rectus fascia can be performed. The lateral distal retractor is put back at its primary position afterward **(Figure 51a, 51b)**.

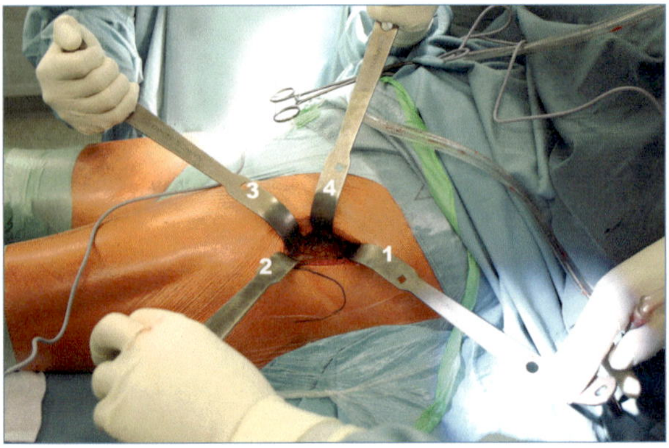

Figure 51a

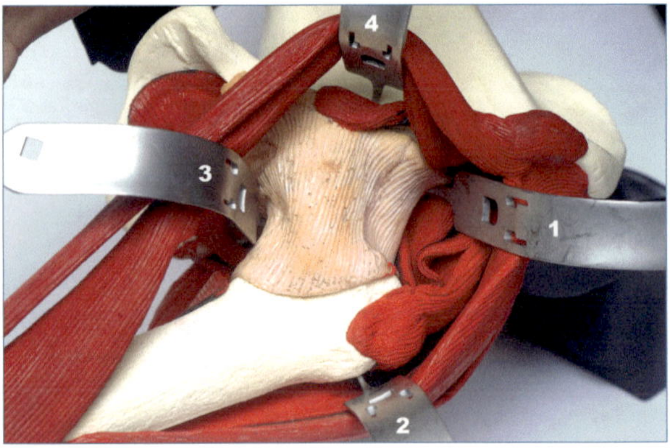

Figure 51b

Injuries to the femoral nerve or the vascular bundle may be avoided if the retractor is placed perpendicular to the ilioinguinal band and kept under the ilipsoas muscle **(Figure 52)**.

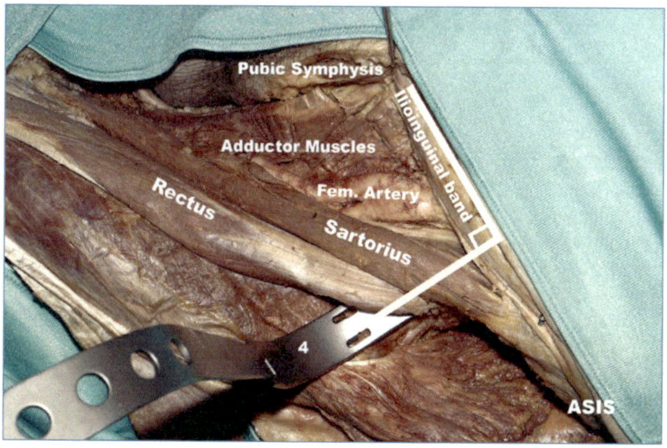

Figure 52

The Portal and Exposure of the Joint: Summary of Key Steps

- Place the patient in a supine position.
- Identify the ASIS as the center of the coordinate system.
- Start the incision 1.5cm distally and 2 to 3cm laterally to the ASIS.
- Avoid any damage to the fascia.
- Expose the red tensor muscle, perforating vessel and white fascia of gluteus medius.
- Identify the tensor and split its fascia.
- Cauterize the lateral circumflex vessels.
- Use four retractors to expose the hip joint.

Preparation of the Capsule

If necessary the reflected head of the rectus can be incised at its capsular insertion. Typically the main portion of the reflected head originates from the bony acetabular rim **(Figure 53a, 53b)**. The capsule is incised along the neck axis **(Figure 54)**.

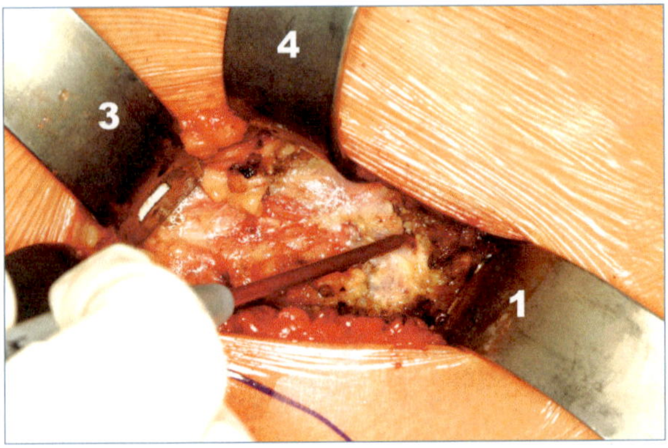

Figure 53a

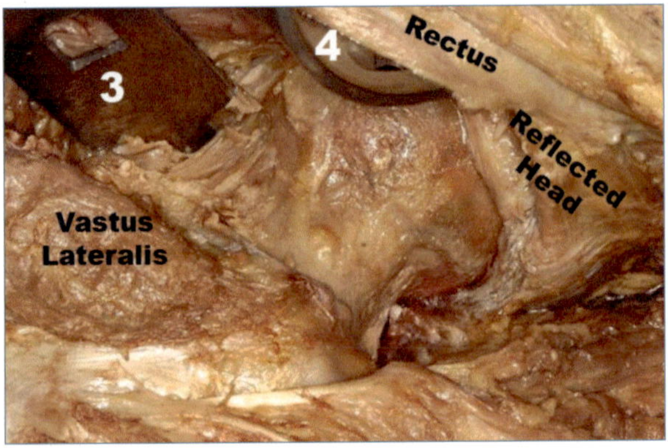

Figure 53b

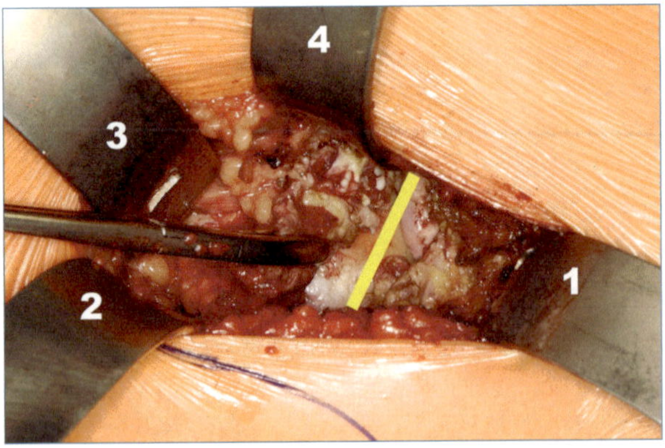

Figure 54

The portion between 11 o'clock and 3 o'clock is removed (ventrolateral flap). If a capsular repair is intended, the flap can be left in place and held back by the medial retractor (3). The medial retractor (3) is placed medially to the neck inside the capsule. Create a lateral flap for further preparation later **(Figure 55a, 55b)**.

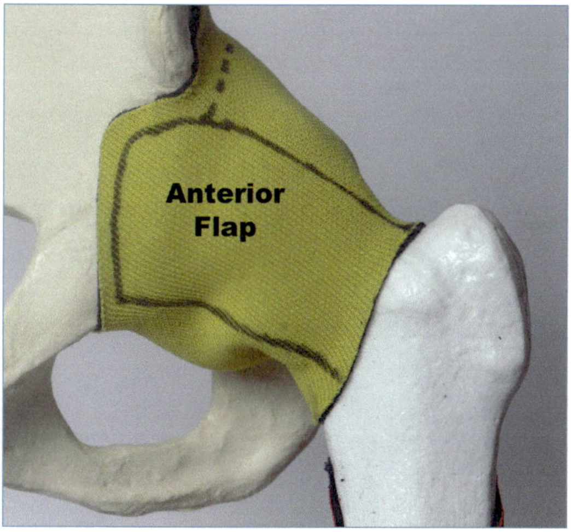

Figure 55a

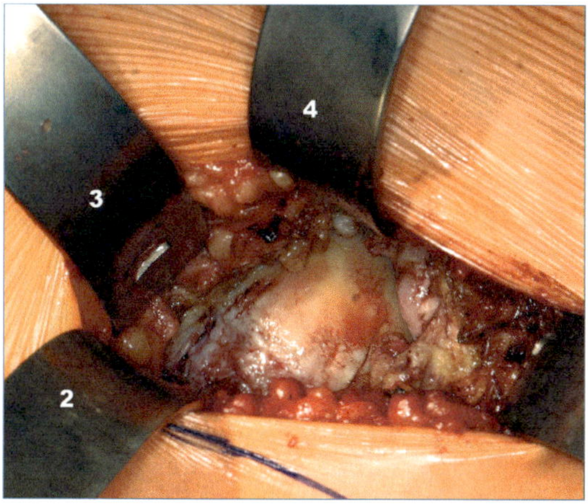

Figure 55b

Carefully clear the "saddle" between greater trochanter and the neck because this is the starting point for the neck osteotomy **(Fig 56a, 56b, 56c, 56d)**.

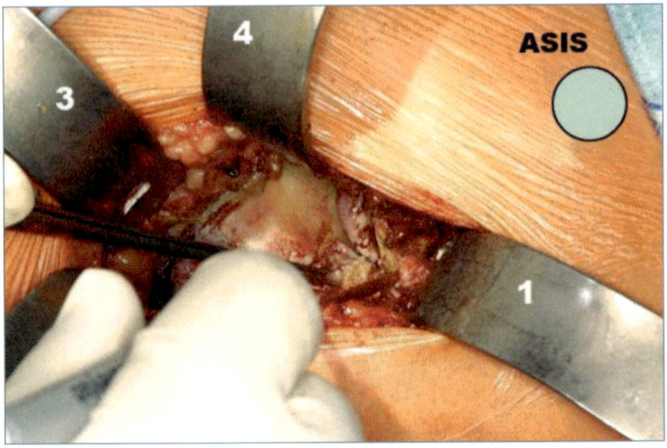

Figure 56a

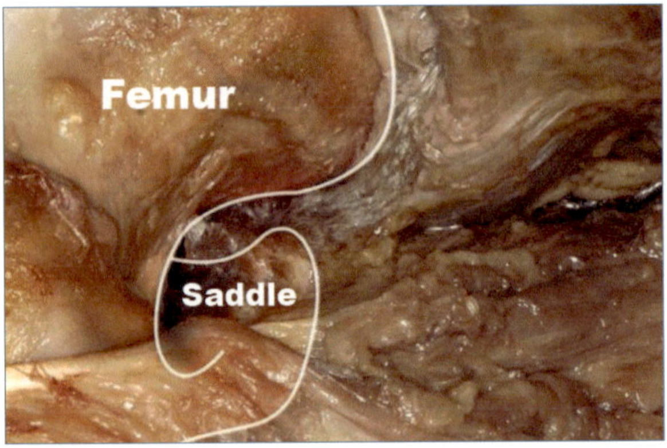

Figure 56b

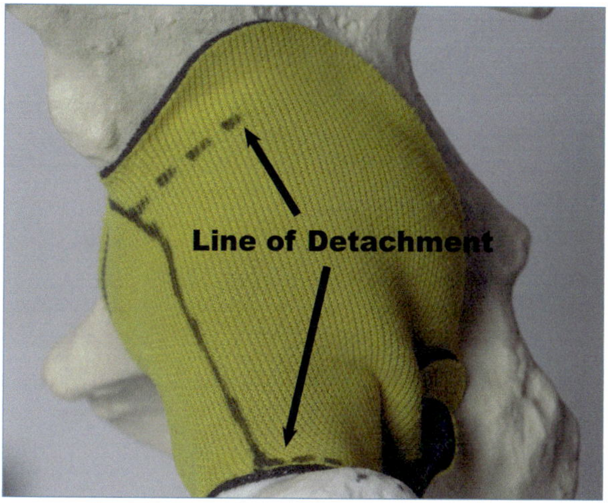

Figure 56c

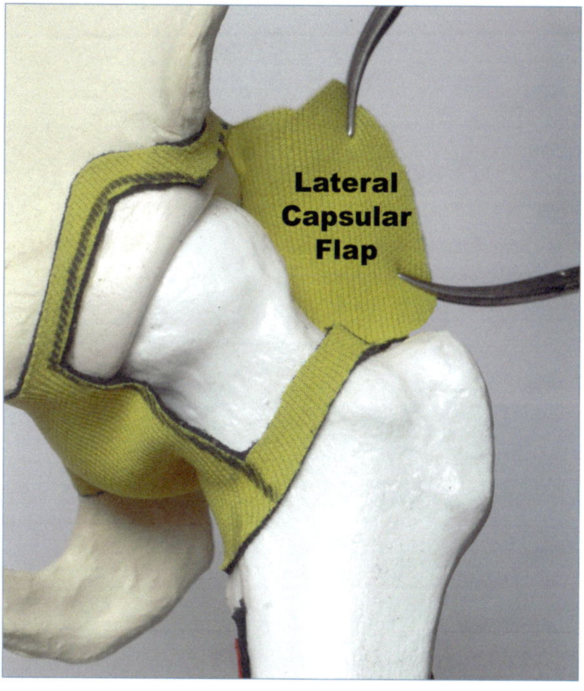

Figure 56d

Osteotomy and the Femoral Head

Remove the supero-lateral retractor (1) and place a blunt retractor (5) intracapsularly in order to protect the tip of the greater trochanter during the osteotomy **(Figure 57a, 57b)**.

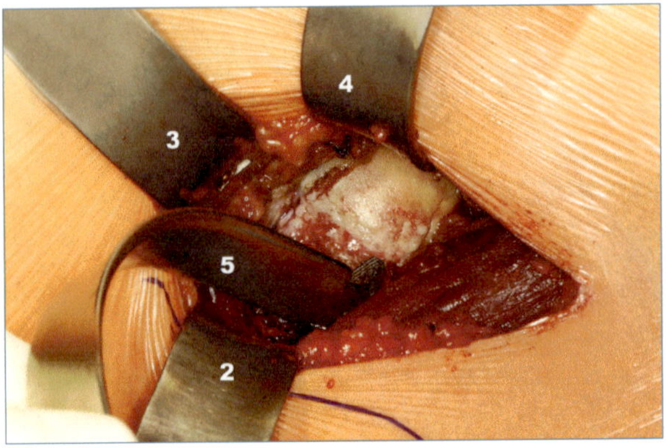

Figure 57a

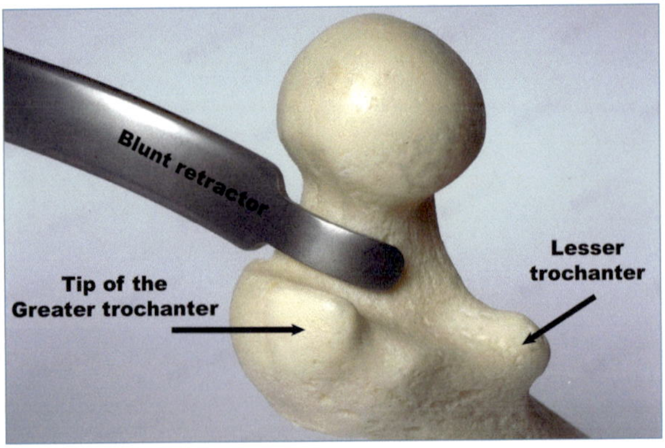

Figure 57b

The osteotomy is based on A/P X-ray planning. The saddle point is used as the starting point **(Figure 58)**.

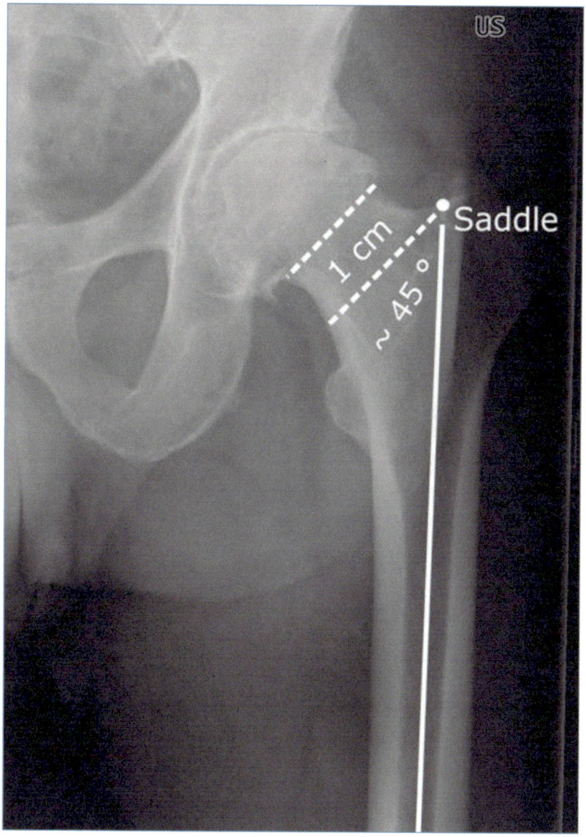

Figure 58

Perform the definitive osteotomy preferably with a small saw that has both a long and small saw blade **(Figure 59)**. Make sure the first osteotomy is complete and perform the second osteotomy on a line from the saddle of the neck approximately 1cm proximally to the first osteotomy. Use the Cobb or a chisel to mobilize the neck disk **(Figure 60a, 60b)**. (Note that the order of the osteotomies can be reversed.)

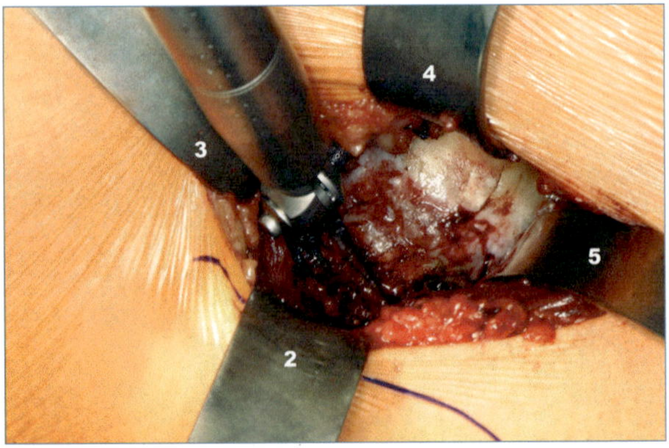

Figure 59

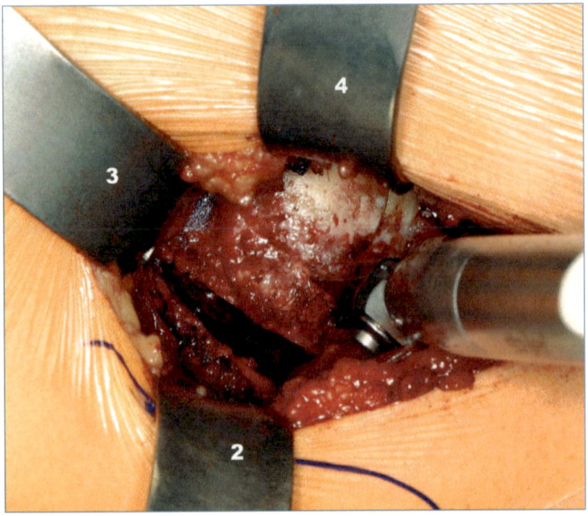

Figure 60a

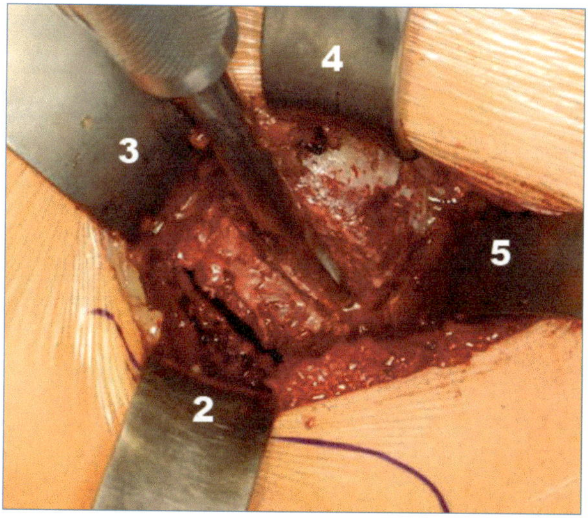

Figure 60b

Remove the neck disk with a clamp or tenaculum. Gentle traction on the leg will facilitate this step. A cork screw is used to remove the remaining head. A gentle but constant longitudinal pull is the recommended technique for removal of the head. Anterior acetabular osteophytes may need to be removed first in order to facilitate femoral head removal **(Figure 61a, 61b, 61c)**.

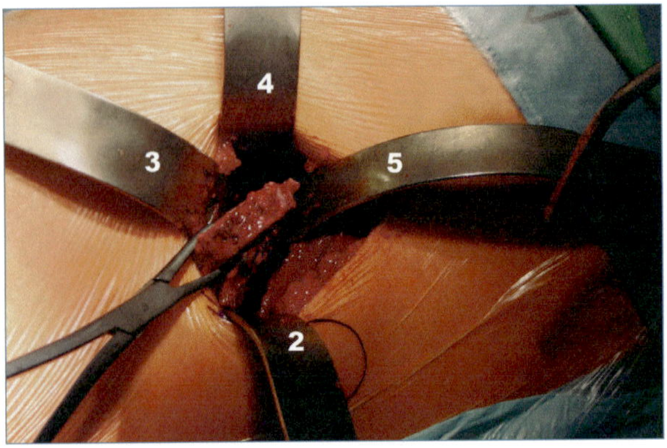

Figure 61a

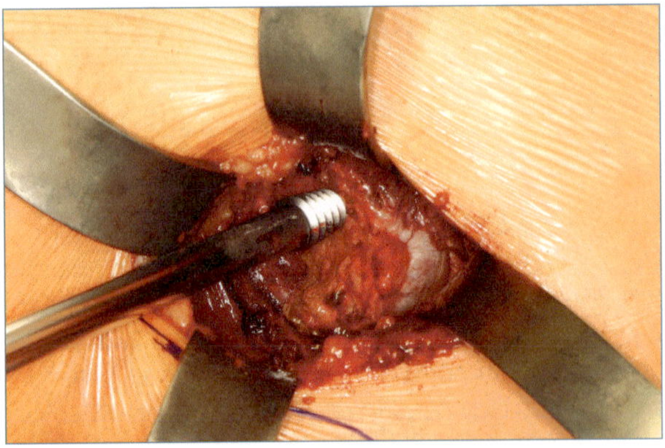

Figure 61b

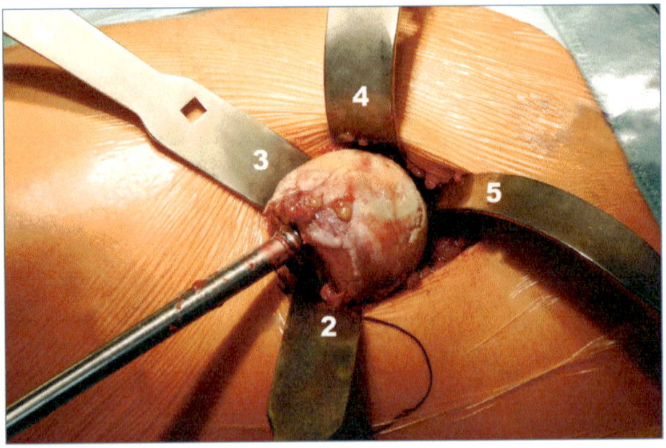

Figure 61c

These steps can be made easier by pulling on the leg in a distal direction **(Figure 62)**.

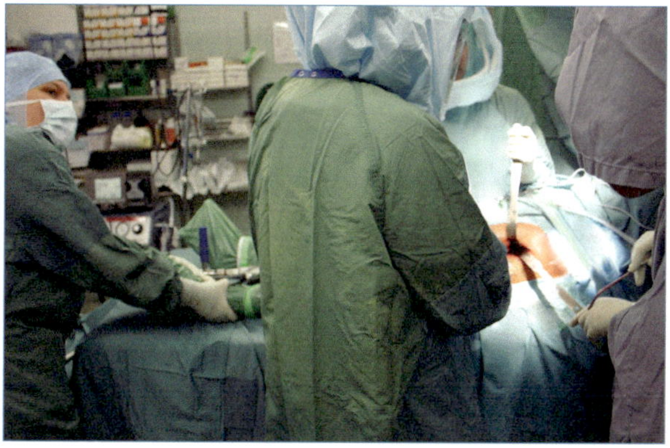

Figure 62

Acetabular Exposure and Preparation

Acetabular Exposure

The ventral retractor (4) is kept in place. Remove all other retractors from their position. A sharp retractor (3) is positioned in the middle of the acetabulum and orientated medially. Scratch along the bone until soft tissue is reached. Now place this retractor around the transverse ligament **(Figure 63)**.

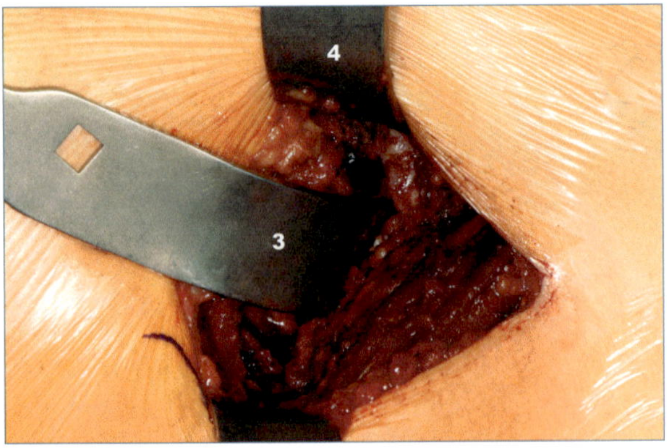

Figure 63

A sharp retractor is placed laterally to the acetabulum (2). Occasionally it is necessary make a small nick in the capsule to facilitate placement of this retractor. At this stage or later, but before acetabular reaming, remove the remaining parts of the labrum **(Figure 64a, 64b)**.

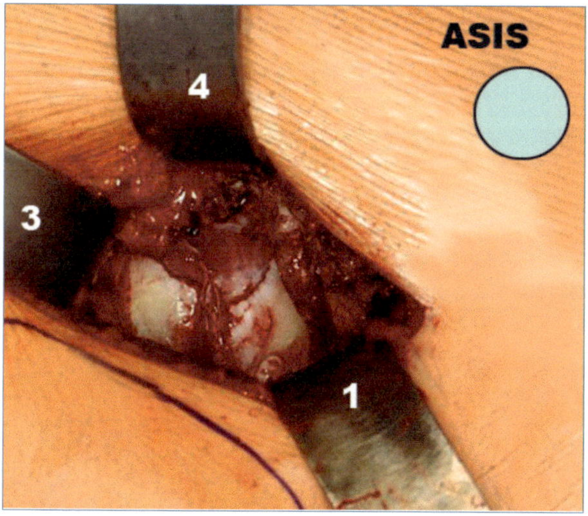

Figure 64a

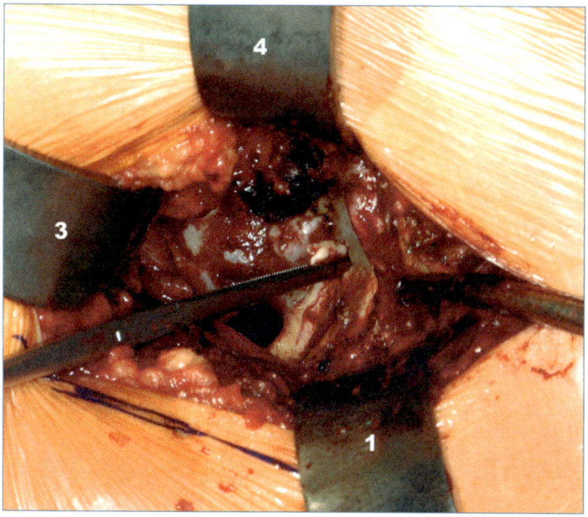

Figure 64b

Preparation of the Acetabulum

Incise the dorsal capsule (it usually forms a roll) in the middle of the acetabulum. Place a double pronged standard Mueller retractor or an acetabular retractor (6) at the dorsal rim of the acetabulum **(Figure 65a, 65b)**.

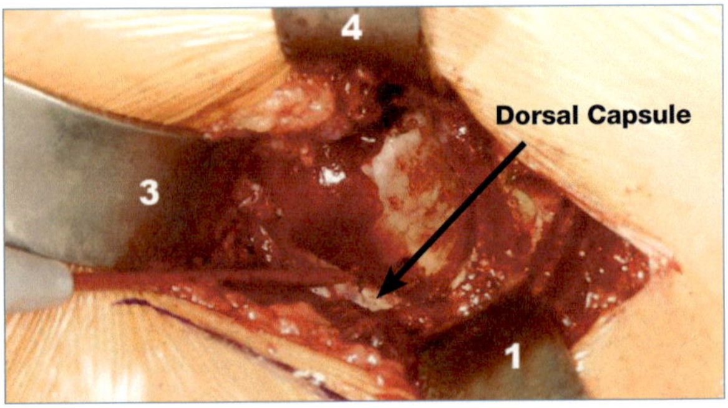

Figure 65a

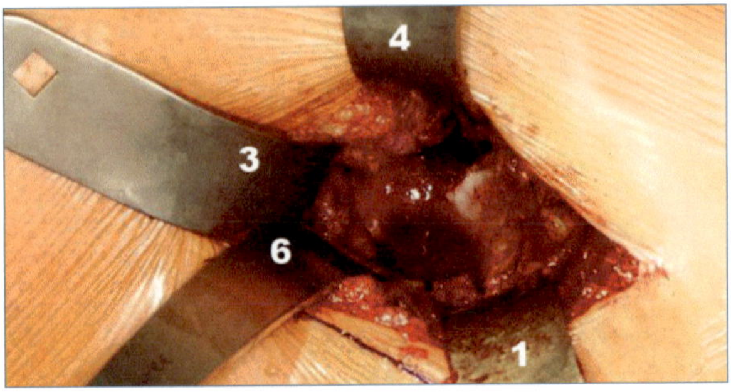

Figure 65b

The retractor can either be held by the first assistant or weights can be used. Ream to the correct size **(Figure 66a, 66b, 66c)**.

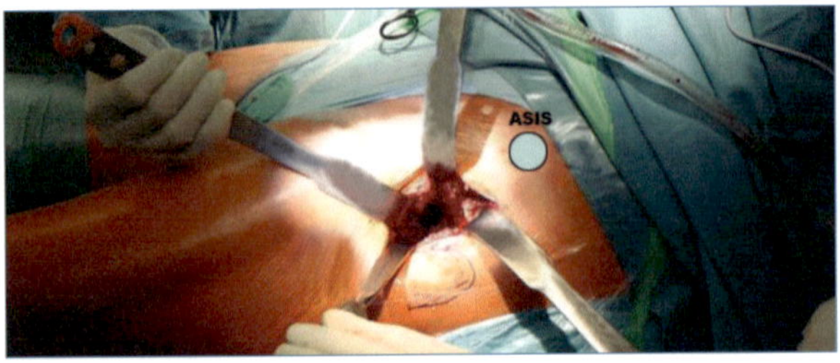

Figure 66a

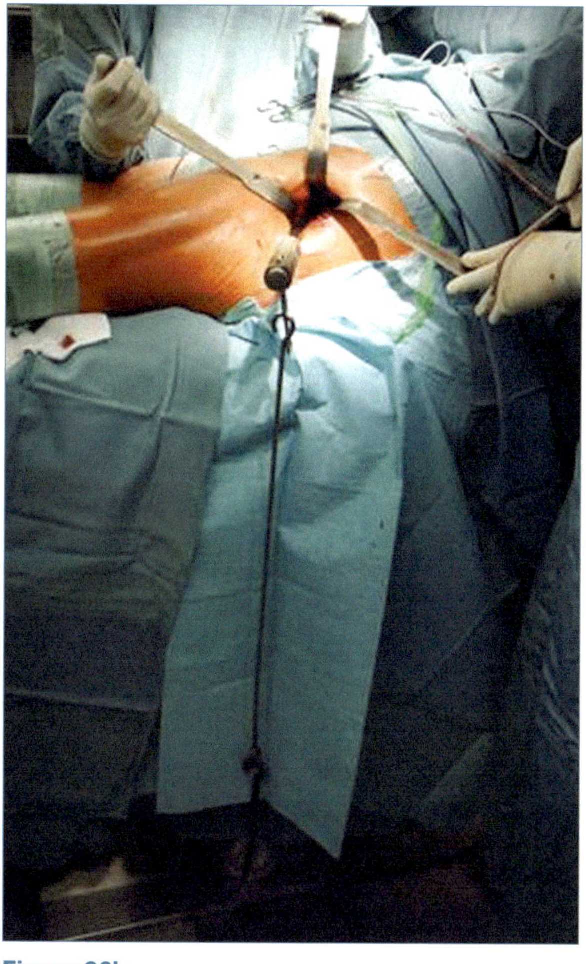

Figure 66b

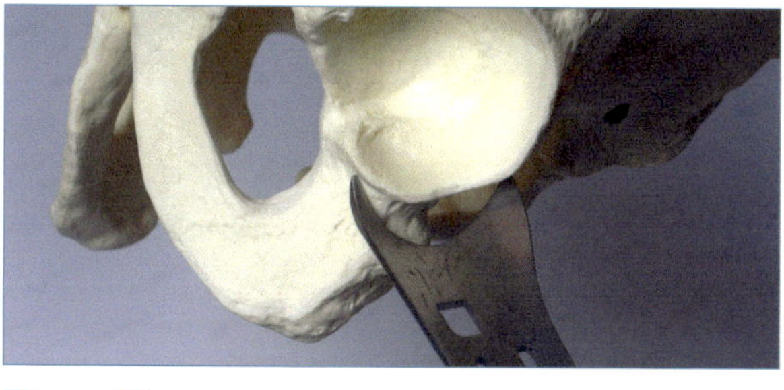

Figure 66c

Method 1: Insert the reamer attached to the reamer handle along the top portion of the retractor. Ream to the correct size **(Figure 67)**.

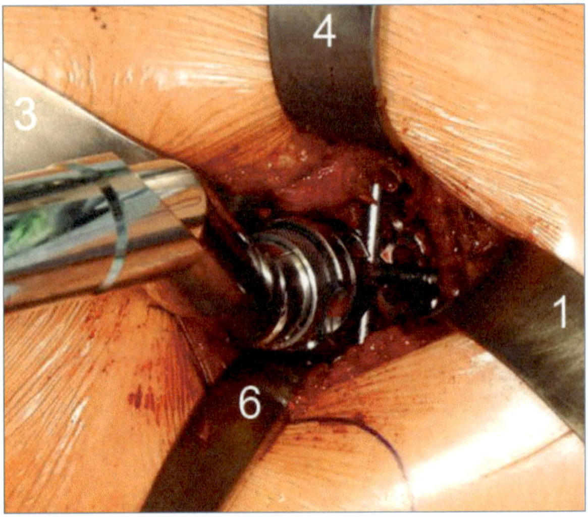

Figure 67

Method 2: In some cases it is easier to insert the reamer and reamer handle separately. In that case, place the reamer in the acetabulum first. Introduce the offset reamer handle and connect it to the reamer **(Figure 68a, 68b)**.

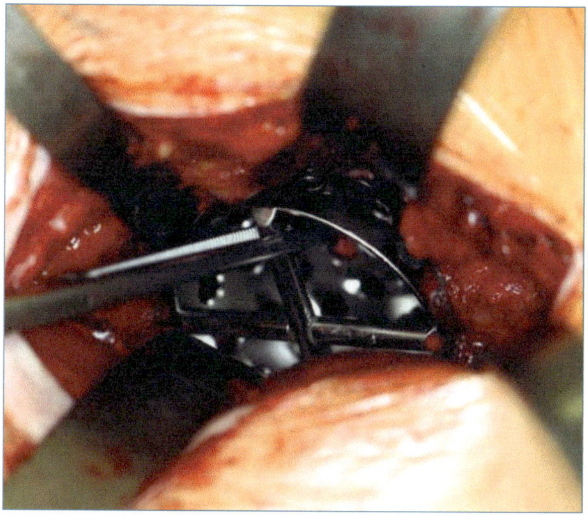

Figure 68a

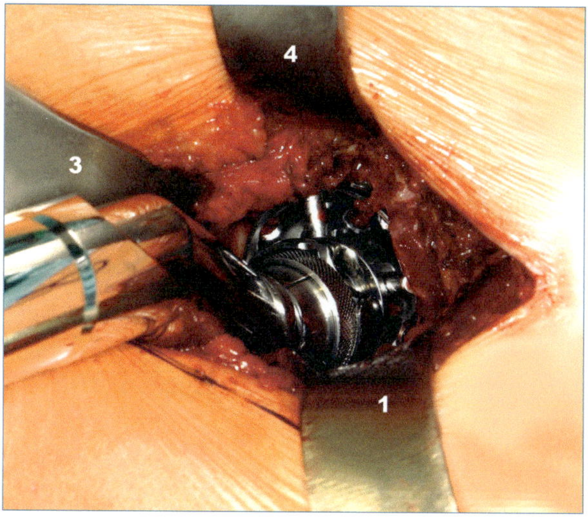

Figure 68b

After reaming, use a clamp to open the locking mechanism of the reamer. The reamer handle is disconnected and removed. Remove the reamer with a clamp **(Figure 68c, 68d)**.

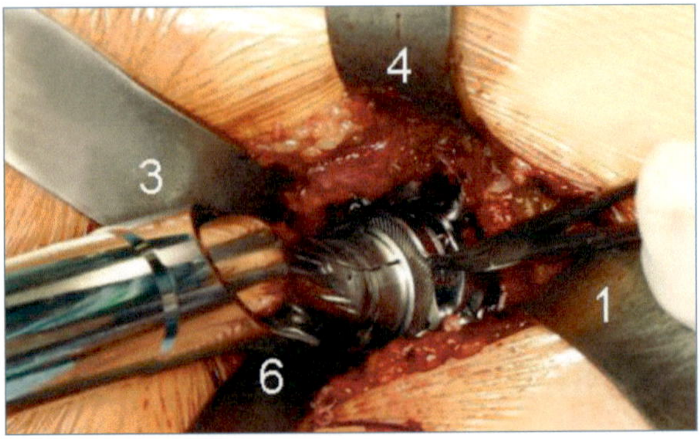

Figure 68c

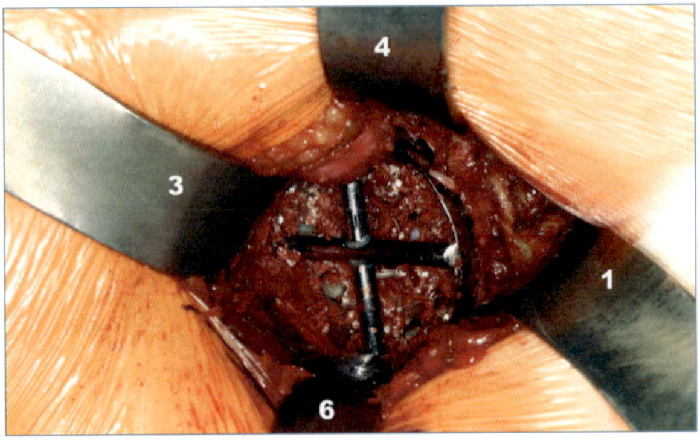

Figure 68d

Cup Impaction

After trialing, use the curved cup impactor to impact the final cup. **Note:** If using a cup with cluster holes, ensure the holes are oriented correctly before impaction, because the cup cannot be re-oriented with the curved cup impactor **(Figure 69a, 69b)**.

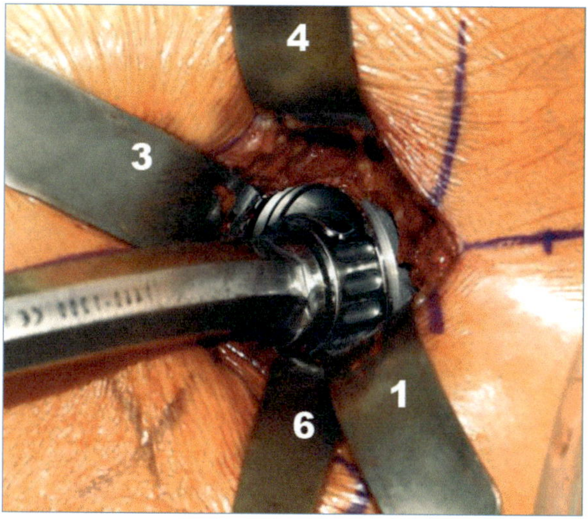

Figure 69a

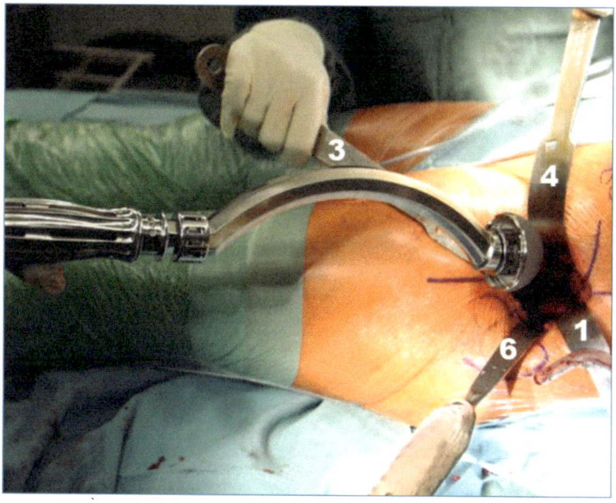

Figure 69b

If the dome hole screw is inserted, use a flexible screw driver or a screw driver with a universal joint **(Figure 70a, 70b)**.

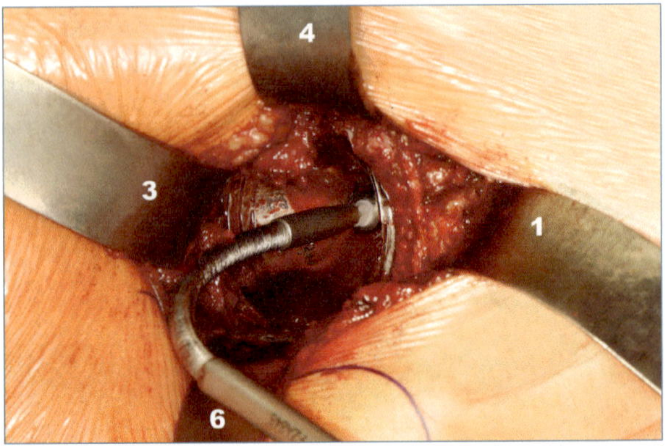

Figure 70a

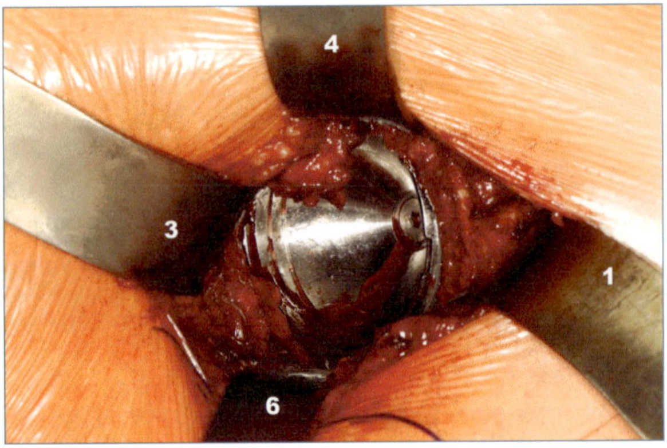

Figure 70b

Cup with Screws

If screws need to be placed, a 90° angulated micro drill is a good option for placing the screw hole in the correct orientation **(Figure 71a, 71b)**.

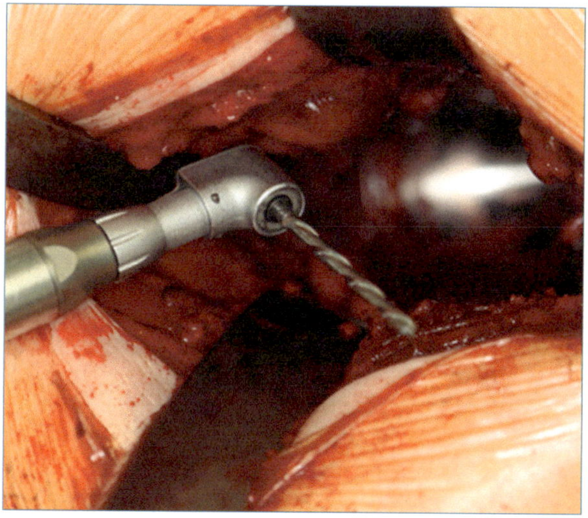

Figure 71a

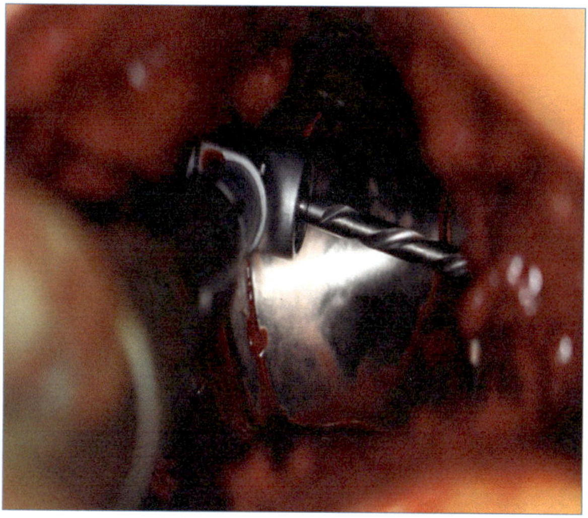

Figure 71b

Use a flexible or a universal joint screw driver to place the screws **(Figure 72)**. Insert the liner **(Figure 73a, 73b)**.

Acetabular Exposure, Preparation, and Cup Impaction: Summary of Key Steps

- Use the saddle point as the starting point for the osteotomy.
- Perform a double osteotomy.
- After removing the head, identify the dorsal capsular roll.
- Remove the osteophytes around the acetabulum before reaming.
- In tight cases, introduce the reamer and reamer handle separately.
- Use an offset reamer handle.
- Use a curved cup impactor.

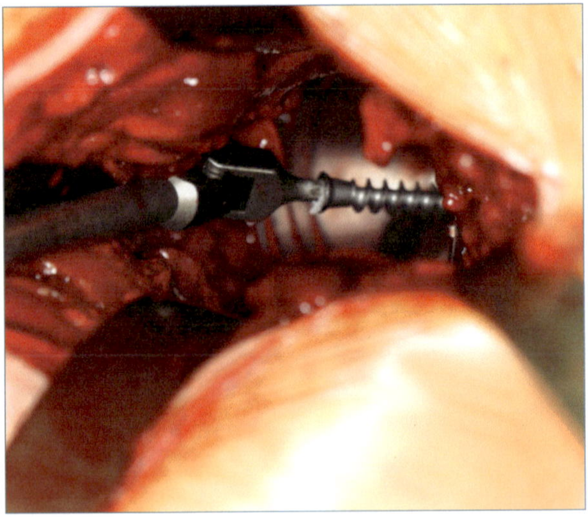

Figure 72

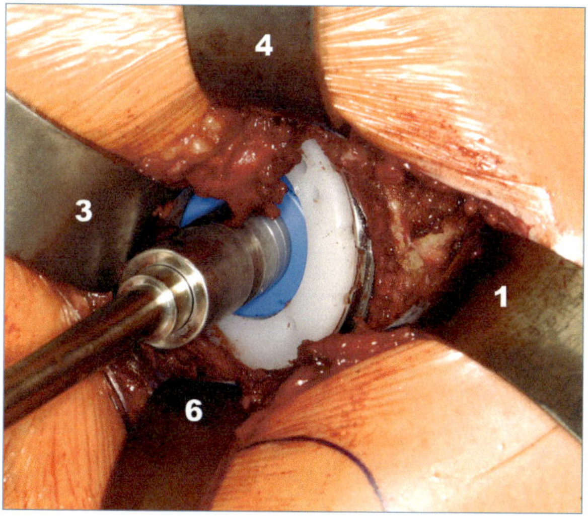

Figure 73a

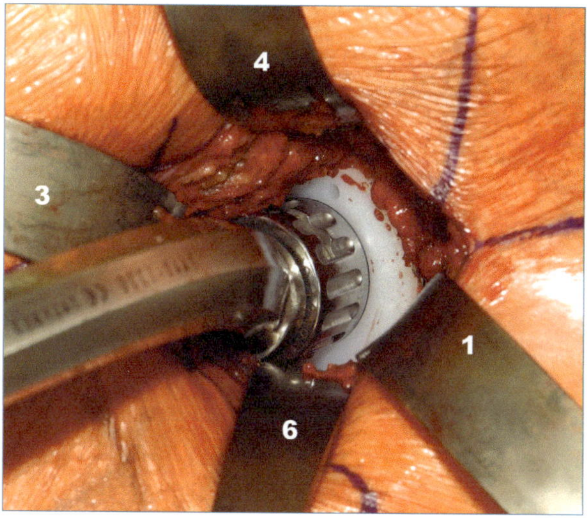

Figure 73b

Preparation of the Dorsolateral Capsule

At this point, femoral preparation will occur. Remove retractors 1 and 6. Put a sharp retractor (1) to the lateral aspect of the greater trochanter. Put the femoral elevator (7) between capsule and external rotator. The lateral capsular flap is grasped with a clamp. Use the electrocautery device to dissect the fat tissue layer between the capsule and the dorsal group of muscles (piriformis, obturator, gemelli) **(Figure 74a, 74b)**.

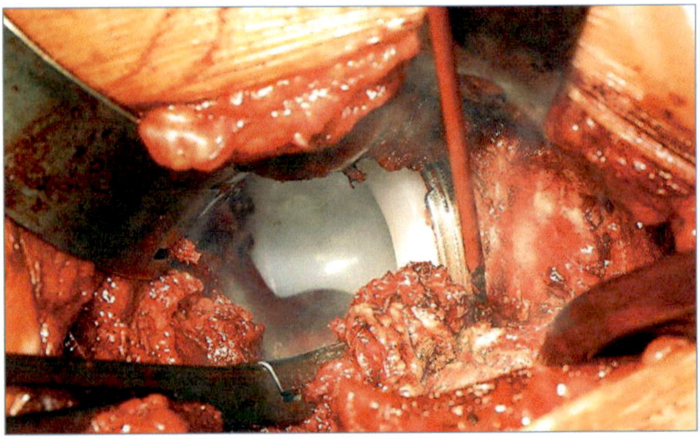

Figure 74a

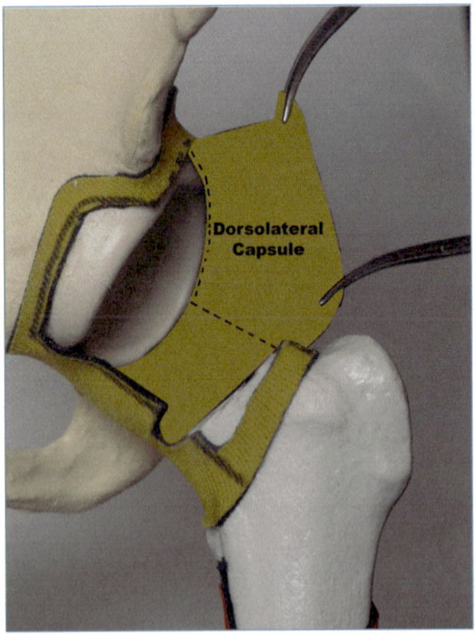

Figure 74b

Figure 4 Position and Femoral Orientation

Remove all retractors and bring the leg in a “figure four” position and place one retractor medially and one laterally to the femur, thus presenting the calcar, which is still covered with capsular tissue **(Figure 75)**.

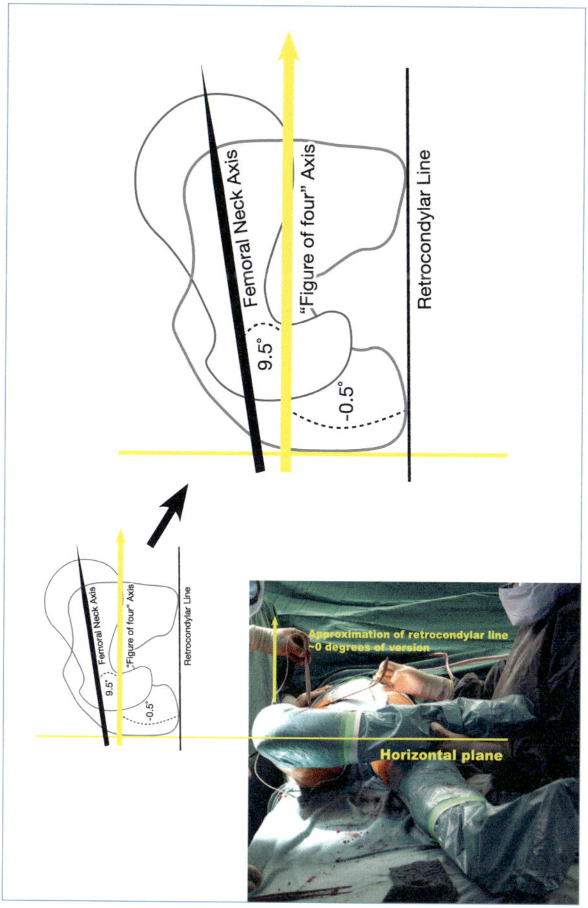

Figure 75. The figure four axis. (For more details, refer to Mayr E, et al. Acta Orthop. 2007;78:458-462.[25])

Use two sharp retractors to expose the calcar. Remove the remaining capsular tissue. If necessary, you can also release the medial and dorsal parts of the capsule in order to improve external rotation. Mark the neutral rotation of the femur with the cautery (according to the "figure four" concept) **(Figure 76)**.

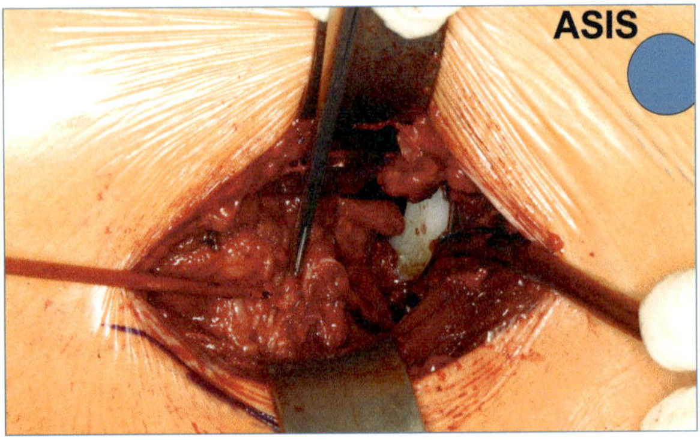

Figure 76

Exposing the Femur

Break the leg part of the table by about 30°- 40° **(Figure 77)**. A custom double pronged retractor (femoral elevator) (8) is placed behind the greater trochanter but in front of the gluteus medius muscle. A bone hook (9) is then placed into the calcar area of the femoral neck. A gradual but firm anterior pull will elevate the femur. The double pronged retractor is then positioned to hold the femur in its elevated position. Additional releases of the posterior structure may be required to achieve proper femoral exposure **(Figure 78)**.

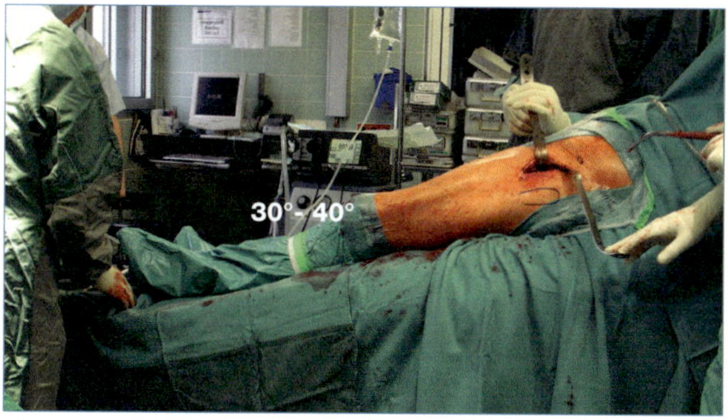

Figure 77

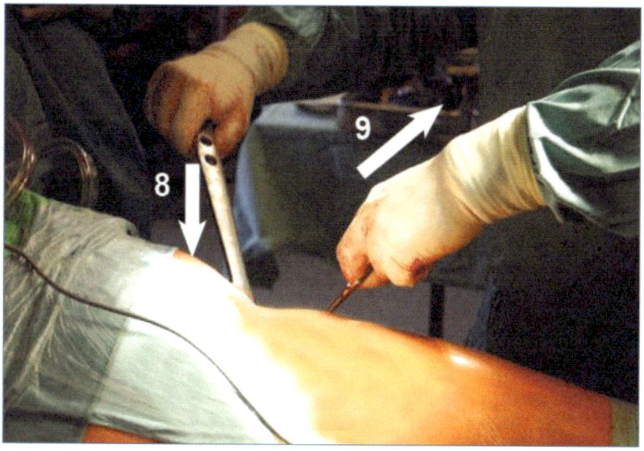

Figure 78

In some cases the tip of the greater trochanter is placed behind the acetabulum. Therefore, pull the bone hook first laterally in order to free the greater trochanter and then pull anteriorly. Always combine pulling the hook and levering with the femoral elevator in order to minimize the forces to the greater trochanter **(Figure 79a, 79b)**.

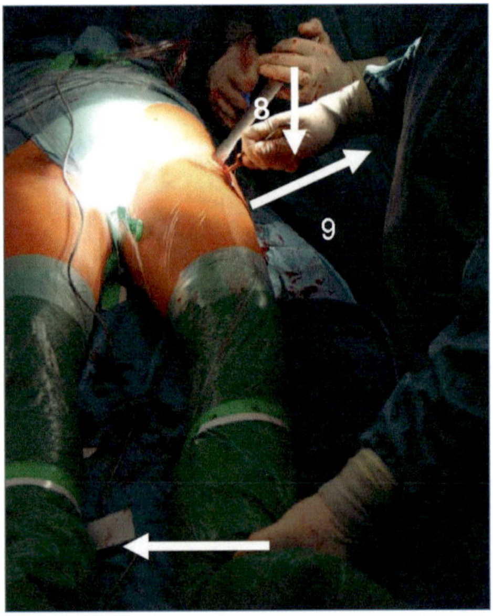

Figure 79a

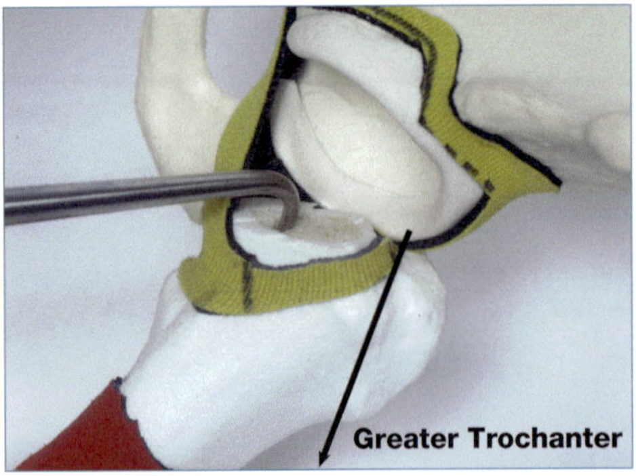

Figure 79b

The opposite leg is abducted and the second assistant externally rotates the leg at the knee. Alternatively, the opposite leg can be crossed over the operated leg and the assistant's hand in order to support external rotation. The operated leg must be placed with a straight knee in order to reduce the muscular force at the proximal femur and to optimize the exposure of the proximal femur **(Figure 80a, 80b)**.

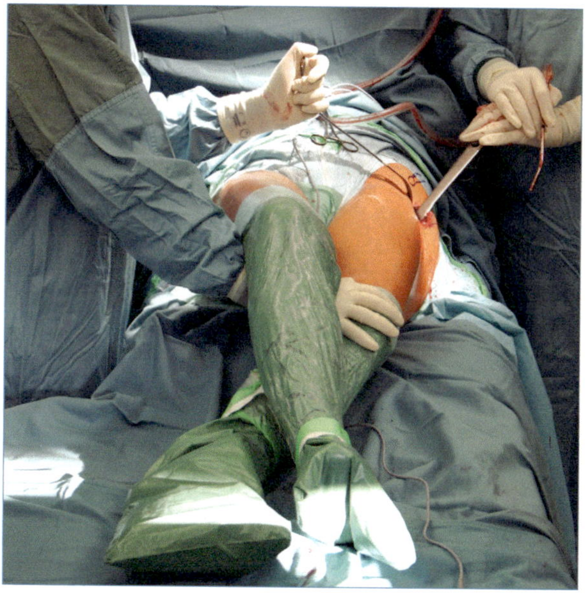

Figure 80a

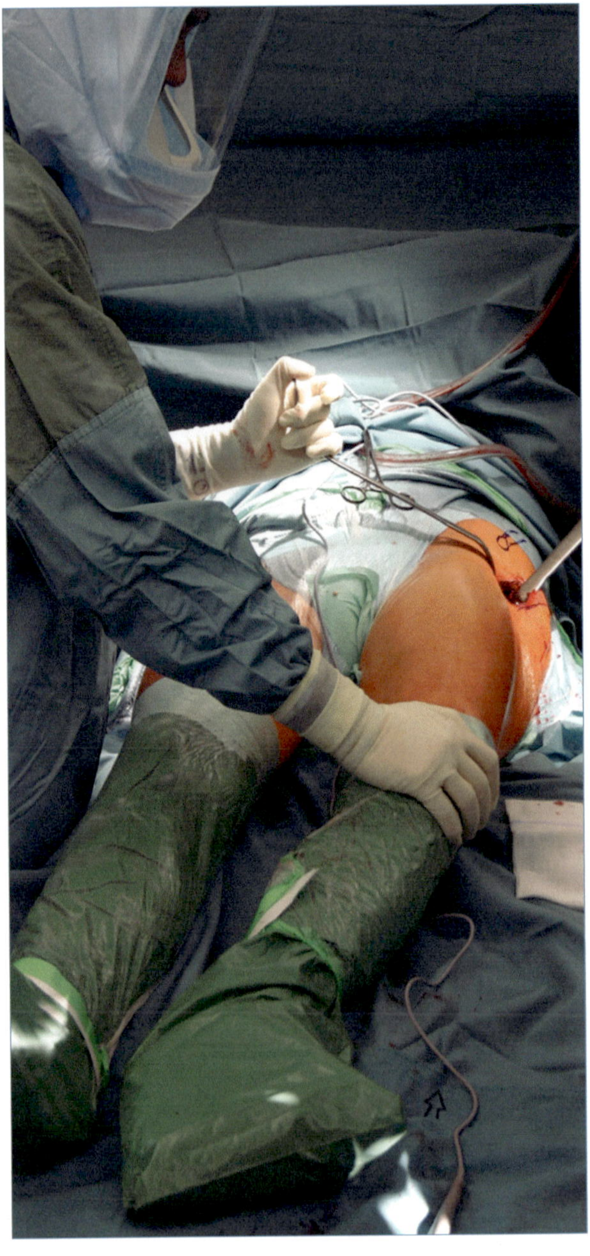

Figure 80b

Possible Releases

The attachments of gluteus minimus, piriformis, gemellus superior, internal obturator and gemellus inferior can be found at the tip of the greater trochanter and in the trochanteric fossa **(Figure 81)**.

Note: There is an optical illusion created by the camera position. In actuality, the bone is recessing within the wound. Also, all instruments must be introduced in a curved manner **(Figure 82a, 82b)**.

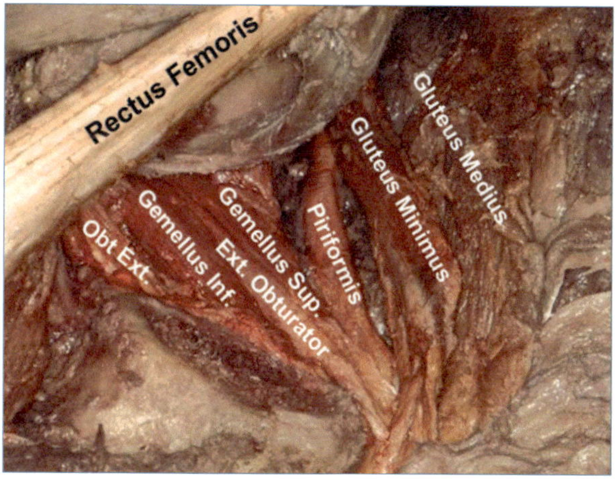

Figure 81

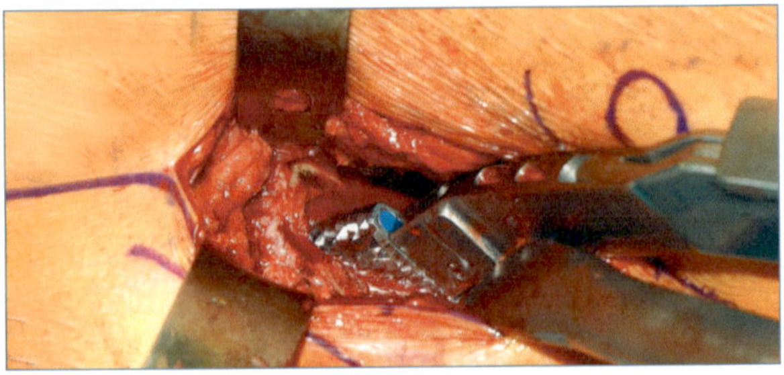

Figure 82a

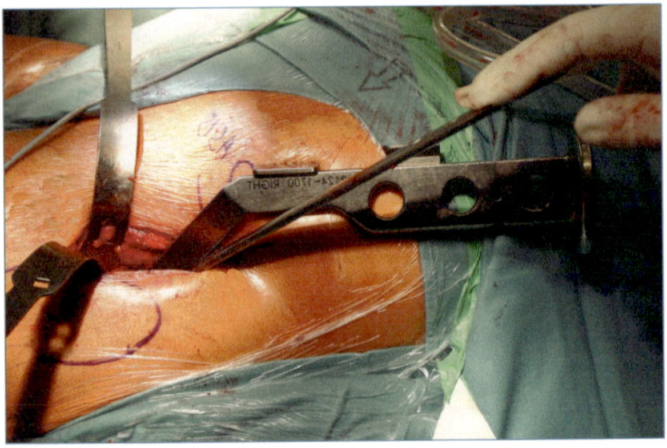

Figure 82b

A sharp retractor (10) is placed at the calcar area proximal to the iliopsoas tendon. Additionally, another sharp retractor (11) can be placed laterally at the proximal femur in order to pull back the lateral soft tissue. After exposing the femur, releases of the above mentioned tendons can be performed if necessary. Even partial release of the joint tendon may significantly increase the amount of elevation you can achieve **(Figure 83a, 83b)**.

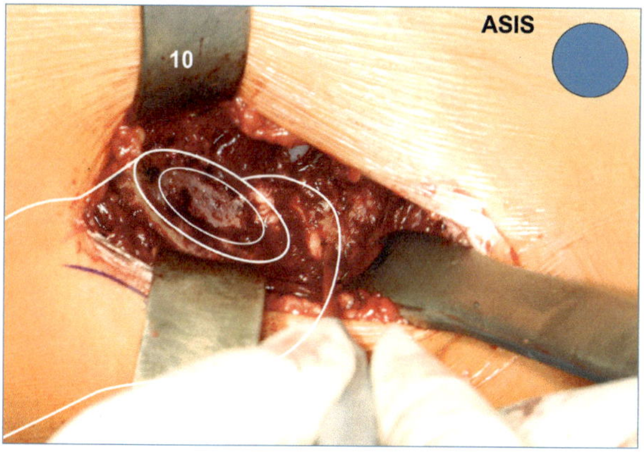

Figure 83a

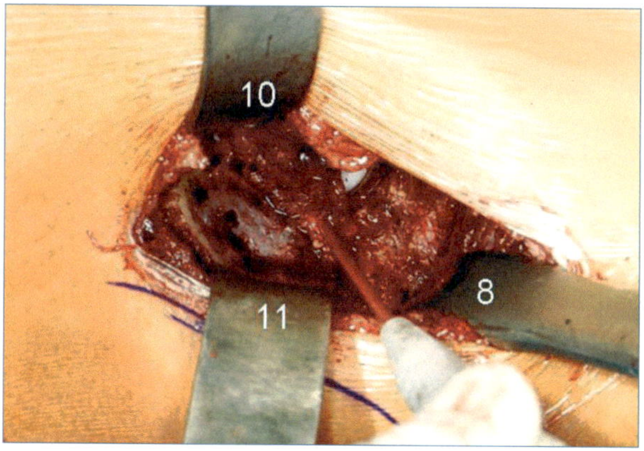

Figure 83b

For Beginners:

A fundamental principle of the muscle sparing philosophy of this technique is to keep all muscles untouched. Yet, especially at the beginning of your experience with the DAA, it is suggested you consider release of these tendons in order to improve the exposure and ameliorate the difficulties of the femoral preparation.

In cases where entering the femoral canal is extremely difficult due to muscle contractures, anatomic variations, or prior surgeries, it is possible to extend the approach proximally **(Figure 84a, 84b)**. Extend the skin incision to the level of the ASIS and expose the origin of the TFL muscle. Release about 1/3 (1 to 1.5cm) of this origin from the ilium. Perform all previously described steps of the exposure again and you should have straight access to the femoral canal. We do not propose this as a principle component of our technique but suggest its use at the beginning of the learning curve only.

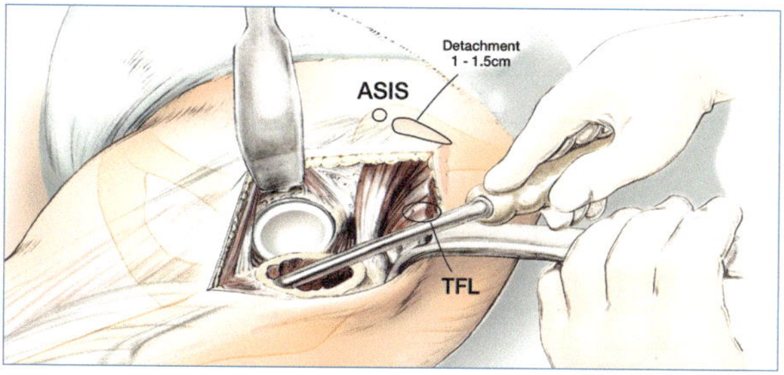

Figure 84a

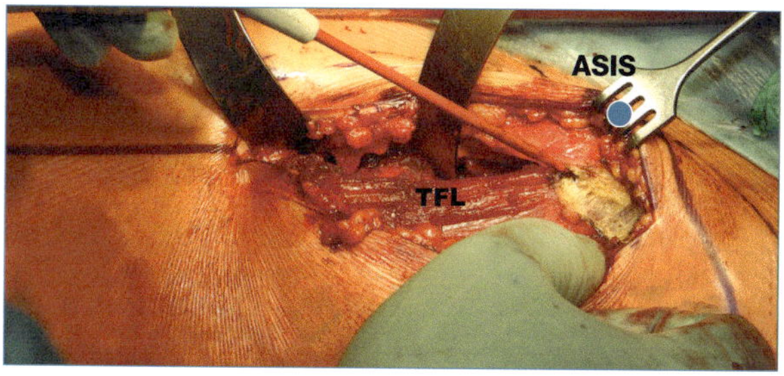

Figure 84b

Preparation of the Dorsolateral Capsule and Exposing the Femur: Summary of Key Steps

- Release of the dorsolateral capsule.
- Hyperextension (break the table).
- External rotation without knee flexion.
- Adduction.
- Femoral retractor dorsolateral to the greater trochanter.
- Femoral hook.

Opening the Femoral Canal and Rasping

Femoral Canal

A curved instrument (i.e., an angulated curette) is used to carefully open the femoral canal and probe it **(Figure 85)**. A rongeur can be used to extend the opening in the direction of the greater trochanter **(Figure 86)**.

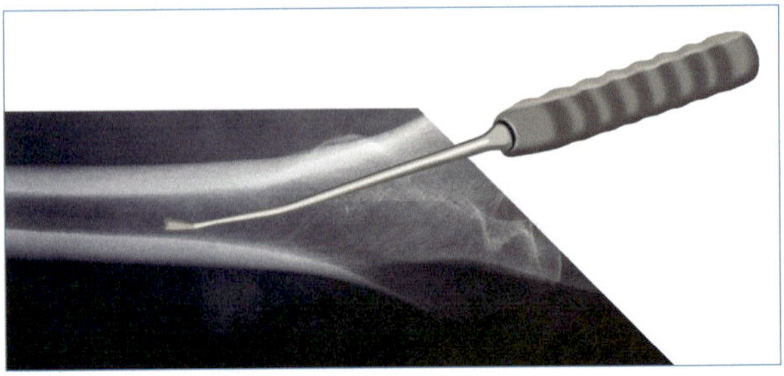

Figure 85

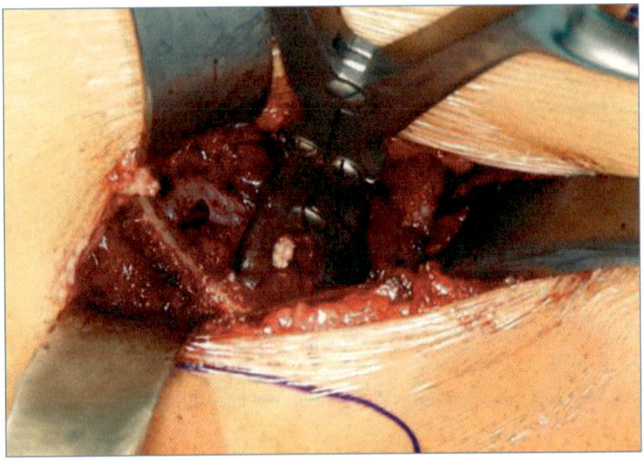

Figure 86

Note: The cortical bone you see laterally to the cut surface is the cortex of the neck and needs to be removed in order to reach the lateral portion of the trochanter (see lateral line along cortex) **(Figure 87)**. A proximal starter broach is used to form the proximal canal **(Figure 88)**.

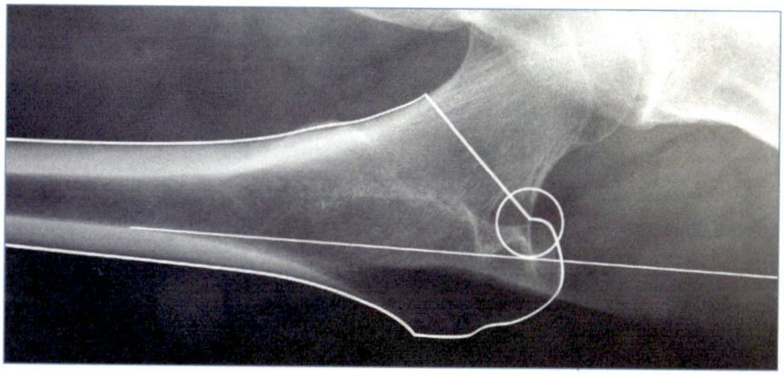

Figure 87

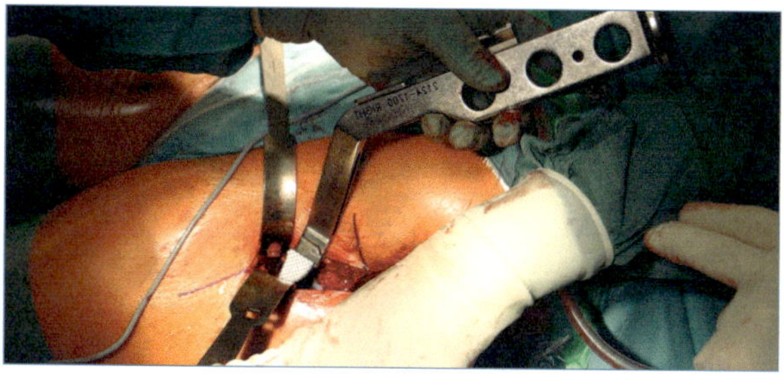

Figure 88

Broaching the Femur

Use the smallest broach available on the double offset broach handle. Carefully slide it along the femoral elevator into the canal. Support the manual introduction by oscillating up and down movements until the broach is perfectly aligned with the femoral canal **(Figure 89a)**. Use the mallet only for the last centimeter of introduction (if necessary at all) **(Figure 89b, 89c, 89d)**.

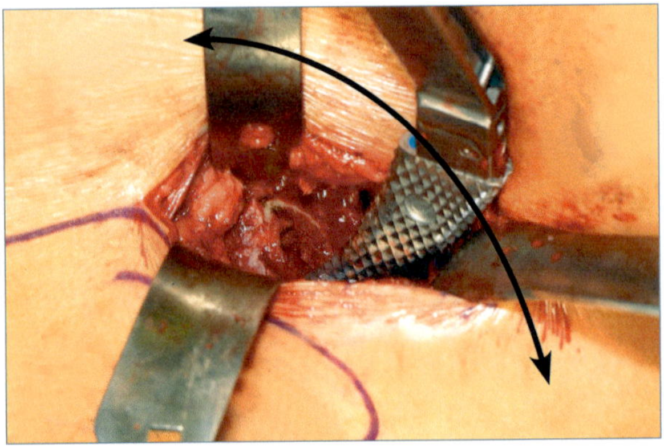

Figure 89a

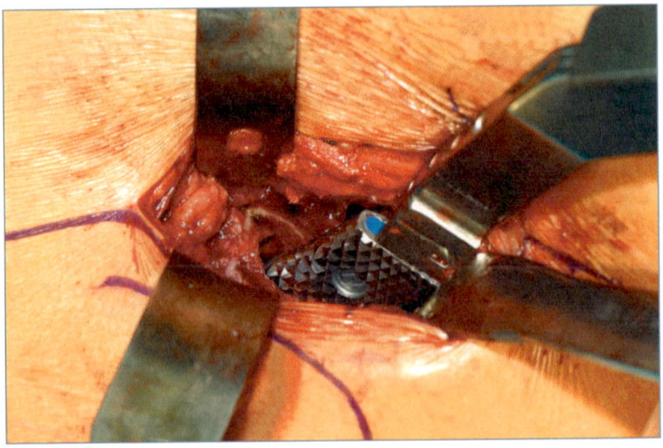

Figure 89b

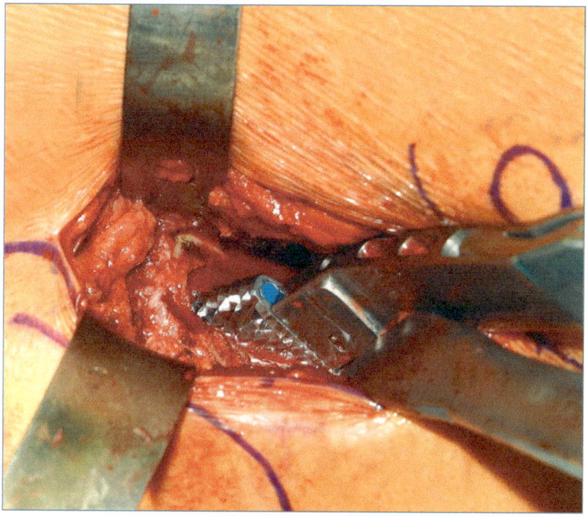

Figure 89c

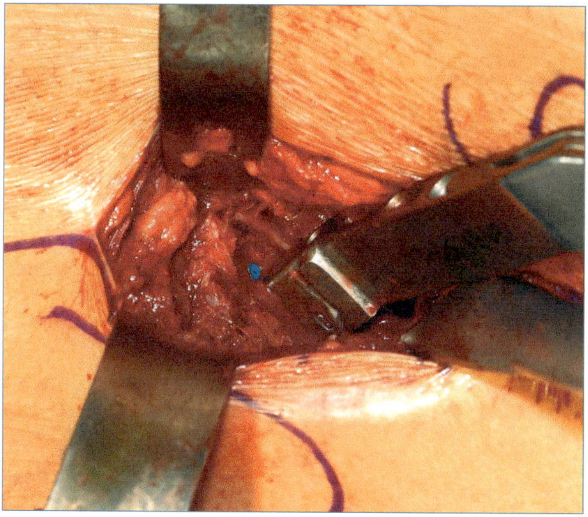

Figure 89d

When you start the manual introduction, initially the broach will be in varus. With oscillating movements, push in the broach until the handle is parallel to the femoral canal. The broach handle should always be medial to the femoral elevator **(Figure 90a, 90b, 90c)**.

Note: In some cases, particularly in muscular patients, less than maximum adduction may provide better exposure **(Figure 91)**.

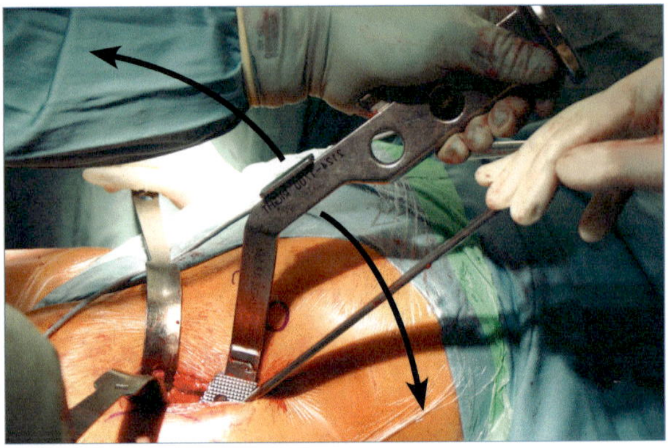

Figure 90a

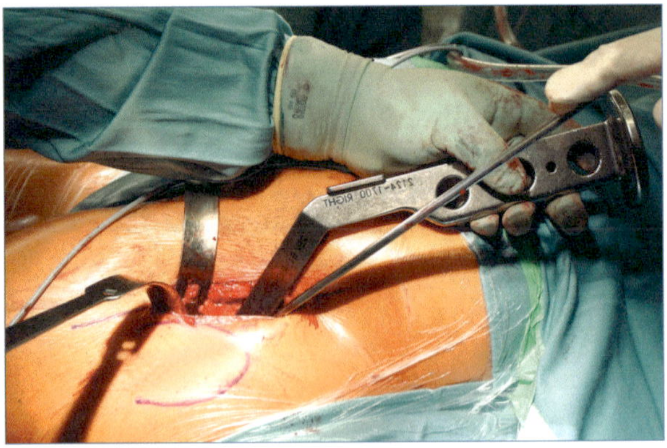

Figure 90b

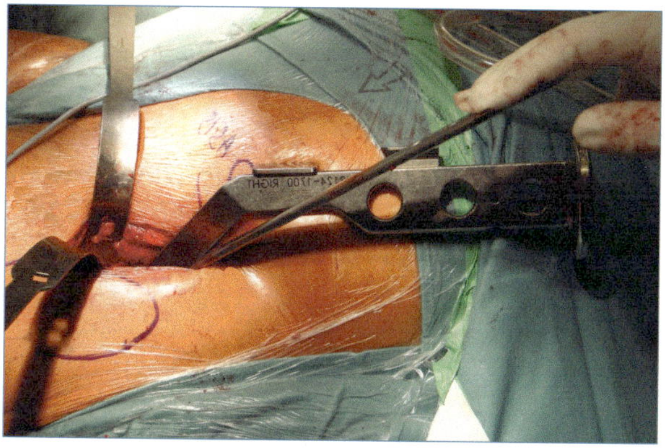

Figure 90c

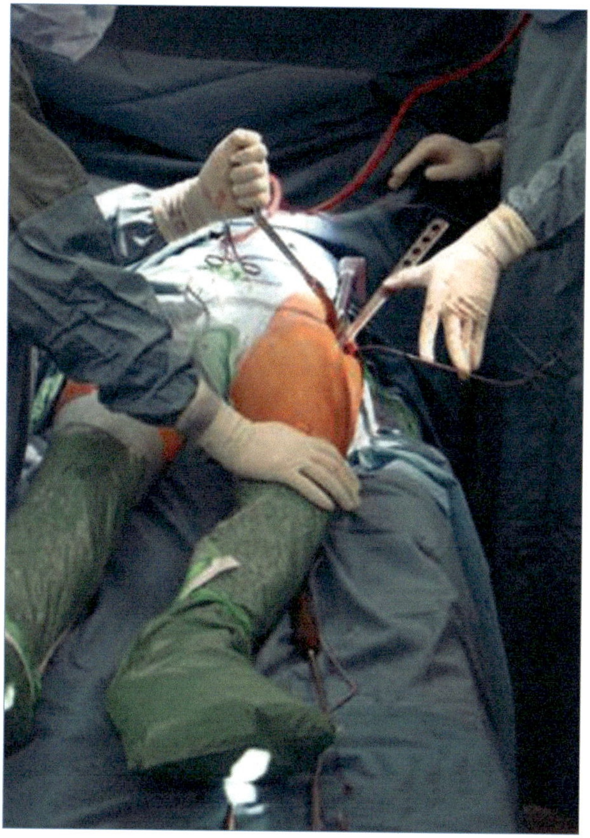

Figure 91

Use the curette to remove debris after each broaching step and also use it to carve out cancellous bone in order to guarantee maximum lateral alignment of the stem **(Figure 92a)**. Probing with a flexible probe allows you to check for accidental perforations as well as the orientation of the direction of the femoral canal **(Figure 92b)**.

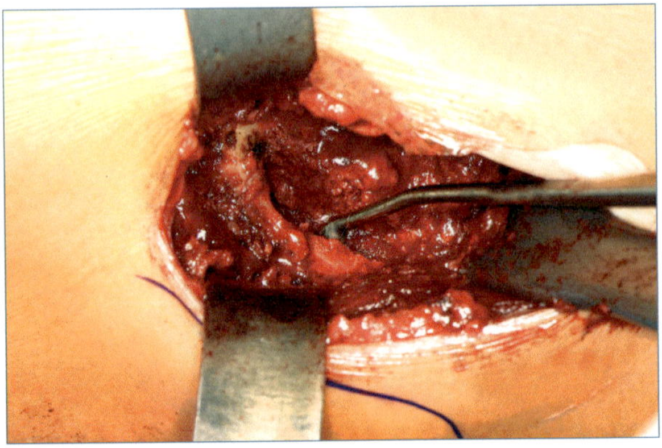

Figure 92a

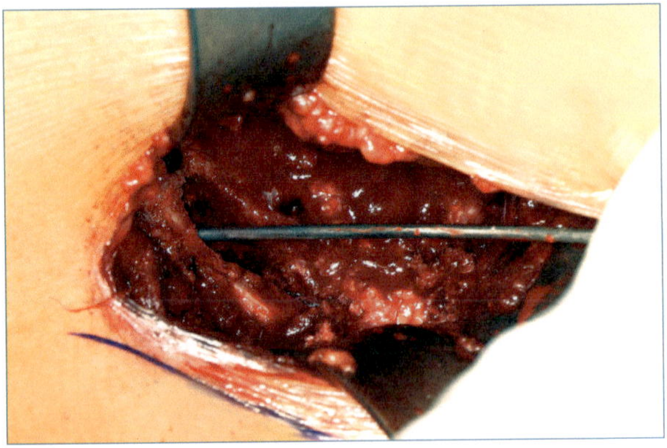

Figure 92b

Implantation and Closure

The final implant is introduced by hand and then impacted gently into the canal **(Figure 93)**. A straight impactor cannot be used in the standard fashion. Rather, it should be placed into the femoral stem impaction hole at a 30 to 45 degree angle to ensure lateralization of the femoral component and minimize the chance of a medial calcar fracture. Alternatively, a custom angled impactor can be employed. The final head is attached and the hip joint is reduced **(Figure 94)**.

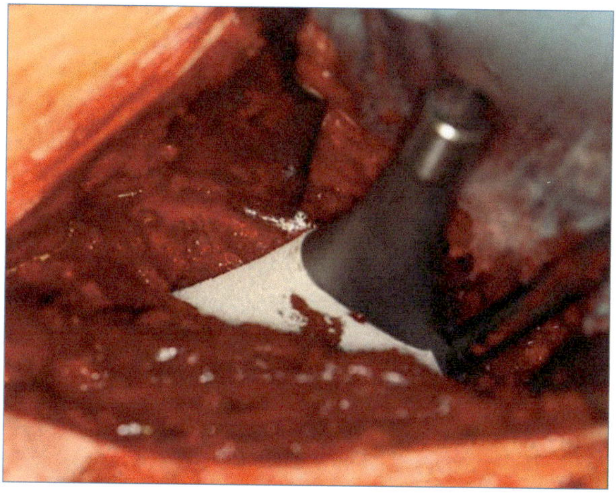

Figure 93

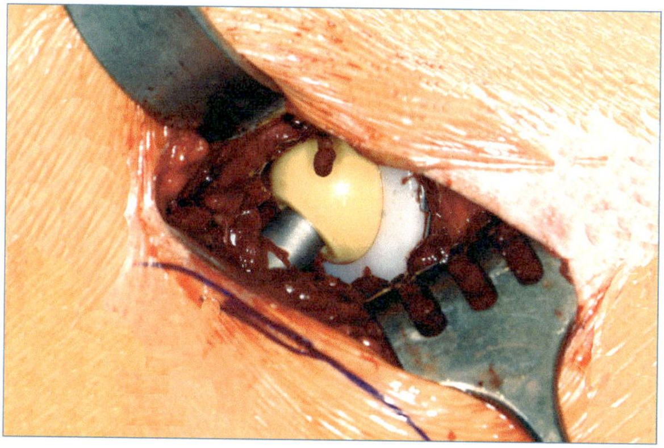

Figure 94

The muscular fascia is sutured. Care is taken to avoid placing suture too far medially—remember, the LFC nerve is there **(Figure 95a, 95b)**.

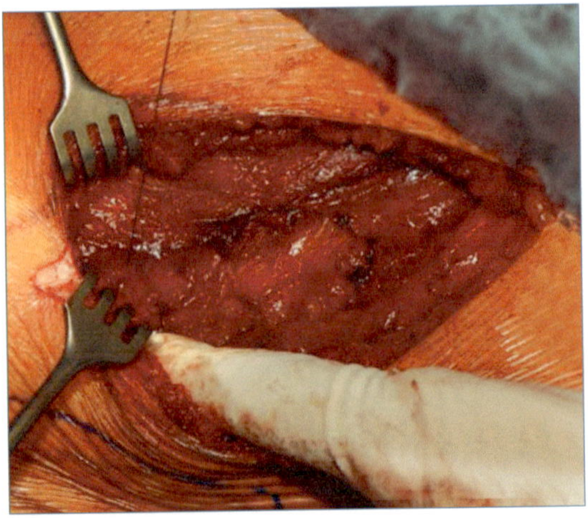

Figure 95a

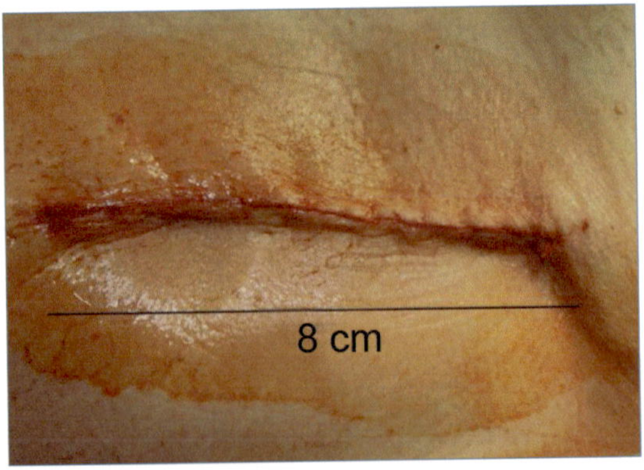

Figure 95b

Opening the Femoral Canal and Implantation: Summary of Key Steps

- Open the femoral canal.
- Manually introduce the broaches.
- Start with the smallest broach handle available.
- Use the double offset broach handle.

REFERENCES

1. Rachbauer F, Krismer M. Minimally invasive total hip arthroplasty via direct anterior approach. Oper Orthop Traumatol. 2008;20:239-251.
2. Light TR, Keggi KJ. Anterior approach to hip arthroplasty. Clin Orthop Relat Res. 1980;152:255-260.
3. Lowell JD, Aufranc OE. The anterior approach to the hip joint. Clin Orthop Relat Res. 1968;61:193-198.
4. Judet H. Five years of experience in hip navigation using a mini-invasive anterior approach. Orthopedics. 2007;30(Suppl 10):S141-S143.
5. Matta JM, Shahrdar C, Ferguson T. Single incision anterior approach for total hip arthroplasty on an orthopaedic table. Clin Orthop Relat Res. 2005;441:115-124.
6. Nogler M. Navigated minimal invasive total hip arthroplasty. Surg Technol Int. 2004;12:259-262.
7. Ropars M, Morandi X. Anatomical study of the lateral femoral cutaneous nerve with special reference to minimally invasive approach for total hip replacement. Surg Radiol Anat. 2009;31:199-204.
8. Nogler M, Mayr E, Krismer M, et al. Reduced variability in cup positioning: the direct anterior surgical approach using navigation. Acta Orthop. 2008;79:789-793.
9. Kolodziej L, Bohatyrewicz A, Zietek P. Minimally invasive direct anterior approach for revision total hip arthroplasty. Chir Narzadow Ruchu Ortop Pol. 2008;73:359-362.
10. Lovell T. Single-incision direct anterior approach for total hip arthroplasty using a standard operating table. J Arthroplasty. 2008;23(7 Suppl):64-68.
11. Siguier T, Siguier M, Brumpt B. Mini-incision anterior approach does not increase dislocation rate: a study of 1,037 total hip replacements. Clin Orthop Relat Res. 2004;426:164-173.
12. Paillard P. Hip replacement by a minimal anterior approach. Int Orthop. 2007;31(Suppl 1):S13-S15.
13. Nogler M, Krismer M, Hozack WJ, et al. A double offset broach handle for preparation of the femoral cavity in minimally invasive direct anterior total hip arthroplasty. J Arthroplasty. 2006;21:1206-1208.

14. Senn N. Tuberculosis of ankle joint and tarsus. In: Tuberculosis of Bones and Joints. Philadelphia, PA: FA Davis Publishers; 1893;473-476.
15. Smith-Petersen MN. Approach to and exposure of the hip joint for mold arthroplasty. J Bone Joint Surg Am. 1949;31A:40-46.
16. Smith-Petersen MN. Evolution of mould arthroplasty of the hip joint. J Bone Joint Surg Br. 1948;30B:59-75.
17. Judet R, Judet J. Technique and results with the acrylic femoral head prosthesis. J Bone Joint Surg Br. 1952;34:173-180.
18. Judet J, Judet R. The use of an artificial femoral head for arthroplasty of the hip joint. J Bone Joint Surg Br. 1950;32B:166-173.
19. Wagner H. Surface replacement arthroplasty of the hip. Clin Orthop Relat Res. 1978;441:134:102-130.
20. Kennon R, Keggi J, Keggi KJ. The anterior approach to hip arthroplasty: the short, single minimally invasive incision. Operative Tech in Orthop. 2004;14:85-93.
21. Keggi KJ, Huo MH, Zatorski LE. Anterior approach to total hip replacement: surgical technique and clinical results of our first one thousand cases using non-cemented prostheses. Yale J Biol Med. 1993;66:243-256.
22. Siebenrock KA, Gautier E, Matta JM, et al. New technique for a hip arthrodesis using an anterior approach and a ventral plate. Orthopade. 1996;25:140-145.
23. Rachbauer F. Minimally invasive total hip arthroplasty via direct anterior approach. Orthopade. 2005;11:1103-1110.
24. Hozack WJ, Klatt BA. Minimally invasive two-incision total hip surgery: is the second incision necessary? Semin Arthro. 2008;19:205-208.
25. Mayr E, Thaler M, Williams A, Moctezuma de La Barrera J, Krismer M, Nogler M. The figure-of-four axis as a reference to determine stem rotation in hip arthroplasty: what does it really measure? a cadaver study. Acta Orthop. 2007;78:458-462.
26. Kennon R, Keggi J, Zatorski LE, et al. Anterior approach for total hip arthroplasty: beyond the minimally invasive technique. J Bone Joint Surg Am. 2004;86-A(Suppl 2):91-97.

SUGGESTED READING

1. Mayr E. A prospective randomized assessment of earlier functional recovery in THA patients treated by minimally invasive direct anterior approach: a gait analysis study. Clin Biomech. 2009;24:812-818.
2. Masonis J, Thompson C, Odum S. Safe and accurate: learning the direct anterior total hip arthroplasty. Orthopedics. 2008;31(12 Suppl 2):129-134.
3. Nogler M, Mayr E, Krismer M, Thaler M. Reduced variability in cup positioning: the direct anterior surgical approach using navigation. Acta Orthop. 2008;79:789-793.
4. Ropars M, Morandi X, Huten D, Thomazeau H, Berton E, Darnault P. Anatomical study of the lateral femoral cutaneous nerve with special reference to minimally invasive anterior approach for total hip replacement. Surg Radiol Anat. 2009;31:199-204.
5. Nakata K, Nishikawa M, Yamamoto K, Hirota S, Yoshikawa H. A clinical comparative study of the direct anterior with mini-posterior approach: two consecutive series. J Arthroplasty. 2009;24:698-704.
6. Vail TP, Callaghan JJ. Minimal incision total hip arthroplasty. J Am Acad Orthop Surg. 2007;15:707-715.
7. Judet H. Five years of experience in hip navigation using a mini-invasive anterior approach. Orthopedics 2007;30(10 Suppl):S141-S143.
8. Oinuma K, Eingartner C, Saito Y, Shiratsuchi H. Total hip arthroplasty by a minimally invasive, direct anterior approach. Oper Orthop Traumatol 2007;19:310-326.
9. Paillard P. Hip replacement by a minimal anterior approach. Int Orthop. 2007;31(Suppl 1):S13-S15.
10. Meneghini RM, Pagnano MW, Trousdale RT, Hozack WJ. Muscle damage during MIS total hip arthroplasty: Smith-Petersen versus posterior approach. Clin Orthop Relat Res. 2006;453:293-298.
11. Siguier T, Siguier M, Brumpt B. Mini-incision anterior approach does not increase dislocation rate: a study of 1037 total hip replacements. Clin Orthop Relat Res. 2004; 426:164-173.

NOTES

NOTES

Made in the USA
Las Vegas, NV
03 November 2026

57423049R00067